Fitness Community Partnerships

This book describes many of the unique contributions of the Food & Fitness program, including a number of early successes, drawing lessons from efforts to form and maintain partnerships, and from the strategies employed to create structural change in communities. This important study introduces the Food & Fitness community partnerships and their work to increase access to healthy, locally grown food, and opportunities for physical activity, in vulnerable communities across the United States. Established in 2007 and funded by the W.K. Kellogg Foundation, the partnerships are increasing the capacity of communities to participate in policy and systems change to positively affect their health and well-being. The material covered in the chapters illustrates how funders, grantees, and partners can work together to create sustainable change at the neighborhood level to ensure that all children and families are able to thrive. A range of studies are looked at from the various initiatives funded nationwide to evaluation methods and results, and an explanation of the role of philanthropy in community development from the viewpoint of the funders. This book was originally published as a special issue of *Community Development.*

Laurie Lachance is an Associate Research Scientist and Evaluation Director of the Center for Managing Chronic Disease. She has led several large-scale, multi-site chronic disease prevention and management evaluation projects, and utilizes community-based approaches creating opportunities for individual health behavior change and changes in health inequities.

Laurie Carpenter is a Senior Research Associate at the Center for Managing Chronic Disease, experienced in research and evaluation of chronic disease management and prevention programs. She has provided leadership and support for several multi-site projects, with particular experience in collaborative evaluation, community-based public health initiatives, and technical assistance.

Mary Emery is a Professor of Sociology and Community Development at South Dakota State University. Her research focuses on community vitality, social and cultural capital, demographic challenges in Indian Country, and the application of systems theory to community change. Her research and service outreach includes improving evaluation and monitoring tools for community change work, applying the community capitals to asset mapping and development, and assessing the impact of community change work.

Mia Luluquisen is Deputy Director of Community Assessment, Planning, and Evaluation at the Alameda County Public Health Department. She has a long commitment to community capacity building and applied research for social action, providing training and technical assistance in program planning, evaluation research, community health education, strategic planning, and organizational development to institutions and organizations around the world.

Community Development – Current Issues Series

Series Editor: Paul LaChapelle

The Community Development Society (CDS) in conjunction with Routledge/Taylor & Francis is pleased to present this series of volumes on current issues in community development. The series is designed to present books organized around special topics or themes, promoting exploration of timely and relevant issues impacting both community development practice and research. Building on a rich history of over 40 years of publishing the journal, *Community Development,* the series will provide reprints of special issues and collections from the journal. Each volume is updated with the editor's introductory chapter, bringing together current applications around the topical theme.

Founded in 1970, the Community Development Society is a professional association serving both researchers and practitioners. CDS actively promotes the continued advancement of the practice and knowledge base of community development. For additional information about CDS, visit www.comm-dev.org

You can see further details about this series on the Routledge website on http://www.routledge.com/books/series/CDS/

Tourism, Planning, and Community Development
Edited by Rhonda G. Phillips

Community Development Approaches to Improving Public Health
Edited by Robert Ogilvie

Community Economic Development
Edited by Rhonda Phillips and Terry L. Besser

Community Leadership Development
Theory, Research and Application
Edited by Mark A. Brennan

Cooperatives and Community Development
Edited by Rhonda Phillips and Vanna Gonzales

Local Food and Community Development
Edited by Gary Paul Green and Rhonda Phillips

Developing Sustainable Agriculture and Community
Edited by Lionel J. Beaulieu and Jeffrey L. Jordan

Sustainable Rural Development
Sustainable Livelihoods and the Community Capitals Framework
Edited by Mary Emery, Isabel Gutierrez-Montes, and Edith Fernandez-Baca

Innovative Community Change Practices
Edited by Norman Walzer and Sam Cordes

Community Visioning Programs
Processes and Outcomes
Edited by Norman Walzer and Gisele F. Hamm

Innovative Measurement and Evaluation of Community Development Practices
Edited by Norman Walzer, Jane Leonard, and Mary Emery

Innovative Community Responses to Disaster
Edited by Brent D. Hales, Norman Walzer, and James R. Calvin

Rural Wealth Creation as a Sustainable Economic Development Strategy
Edited by Shanna Ratner, and Deborah Markley

Regional Equity
Edited by Victor Rubin

Food & Fitness Community Partnerships
Edited by Laurie Lachance, Laurie Carpenter, Mary Emery, and Mia Luluquisen

Food & Fitness Community Partnerships

Edited by

Laurie Lachance, Laurie Carpenter, Mary Emery and Mia Luluquisen

Routledge
Taylor & Francis Group
LONDON AND NEW YORK

First published 2016
by Routledge
2 Park Square, Milton Park, Abingdon, Oxon, OX14 4RN, UK

and by Routledge
605 Third Avenue, New York, NY 10017

Routledge is an imprint of the Taylor & Francis Group, an informa business

British Library Cataloguing in Publication Data
A catalogue record for this book is available from the British Library

ISBN 13: 978-1-138-64690-2 (hbk)

Typeset in Times
by RefineCatch Limited, Bungay, Suffolk

Publisher's Note
The publisher accepts responsibility for any inconsistencies that may have arisen during the conversion of this book from journal articles to book chapters, namely the possible inclusion of journal terminology.

Contents

Citation Information

The chapters in this book were originally published in *Community Development*, volume 5, issue 3 (July 2014). When citing this material, please use the original page numbering for each article, as follows:

Chapter 1
An introduction to the Food & Fitness community partnerships and this special issue
Laurie Lachance, Laurie Carpenter, Mary Emery and Mia Luluquisen
Community Development, volume 5, issue 3 (July 2014) pp. 215–219

Chapter 2
Philanthropy's role: working alongside communities to support social change
Linda Jo Doctor
Community Development, volume 5, issue 3 (July 2014) pp. 220–226

Chapter 3
Food & Community: the cross-site evaluation of the W.K. Kellogg Food & Fitness community partnerships
Laurie Lachance, Laurie Carpenter, Martha Quinn, Margaret K. Wilkin, Edward Green, Kazumi Tsuchiya, Belinda Nelson, Cleopatra Caldwell, Linda Jo Doctor and Noreen M. Clark
Community Development, volume 5, issue 3 (July 2014) pp. 227–239

Chapter 4
FEEST on this: youth engagement for community change in the King County Food and Fitness Initiative
Diana Rowland Charbonneau, Allen Cheadle, Cristina Orbé, Madeline Frey and Brad Gaolach
Community Development, volume 5, issue 3 (July 2014) pp. 240–251

Chapter 5
Community engagement for policy and systems change
Mia Luluquisen and Lauren Pettis
Community Development, volume 5, issue 3 (July 2014) pp. 252–262

Chapter 6

"Call for Partnerships:" an innovative strategy to establish grassroots partnerships to transform the food and fitness environments
Catherine H. Sands, Sarah C. Bankert, Suzanne Rataj, Monica Maitin and Jonell Sostre
Community Development, volume 5, issue 3 (July 2014) pp. 263–278

Chapter 7

Relationship building: the art, craft, and context for mobilizing the social capital necessary for systems change
Mary E. Emery and Corry Bregendahl
Community Development, volume 5, issue 3 (July 2014) pp. 279–292

Chapter 8

Moving toward and beyond equity: the Food & Fitness approach to increasing opportunities for health in communities
Laurie Lachance, Laurie Carpenter, Martha Quinn, Margaret K. Wilkin and Noreen M. Clark
Community Development, volume 5, issue 3 (July 2014) pp. 293–297

Notes on Contributors

Sarah C. Bankert is Prevention Specialist at Community Health Solutions, Northampton, Massachusetts, USA.

Corry Bregendahl is Associate Scientist at the Leopold Center for Sustainable Agriculture, Iowa State University, Ames, Iowa, USA.

Cleopatra Caldwell is Professor of Health Behaviour and Health Education at the Center for Managing Chronic Disease, University of Michigan, Ann Arbor, Michigan, USA.

Laurie Carpenter is a Senior Research Associate at the Center for Managing Chronic Disease University of Michigan, Ann Arbor, Michigan, USA.

Diana Rowland Charbonneau is Senior Research Associate and Program Manager of the Group Health Research Institute in Seattle, Washington, USA.

Allen Cheadle is Director of the Center for Community Health and Evaluation and Senior Investigator of the Group Health Research Institute in Seattle, Washington, USA.

Noreen M. Clark is Professor of Public Health and Director of the Center for Managing Chronic Disease, University of Michigan, Ann Arbor, Michigan, USA.

Linda Jo Doctor is Program Officer for the W.K. Kellogg Foundation in Battle Creek, Michigan, USA.

Mary Emery is a Professor of Sociology and Community Development at South Dakota State University, Brookings, South Dakota, USA.

Madeline Frey is Director of Evaluation at the Healthcare Georgia Foundation in Atlanta, Georgia, USA.

Brad Gaolach is a Community Sustainability Specialist in the Extension Community and Economic Development Program Unit at Washington State University, Tacoma, Washington, USA.

Edward Green is a Research Area Specialist at the Center for Managing Chronic Disease, University of Michigan, Ann Arbor, Michigan, USA.

Laurie Lachance is an Associate Research Scientist and Evaluation Director of the Center for Managing Chronic Disease, University of Michigan, Ann Arbor, Michigan, USA.

Mia Luluquisen is Deputy Director of Community Assessment, Planning, and Evaluation at the Alameda County Public Health Department, Oakland, California, USA.

Monica Maitin is a research student at Holyoke Community College, Holyoke, Massachusetts, USA.

Belinda Nelson is Research Investigator at the Center for Managing Chronic Disease, University of Michigan, Ann Arbor, Michigan, USA.

Cristina Orbé is Executive Director of FEEST in Seattle, Washington, USA.

Lauren Pettis is a researcher at the Alameda County Public Health Department, Oakland, California, USA.

Martha Quinn is Research Area Specialist at the Center for Managing Chronic Disease, University of Michigan, USA.

Suzanne Rataj is Evaluation Manager at the Department of Public Health, University of Massachusetts, Amherst, Massachsetts, USA.

Catherine H. Sands is a Lecturer at U Mass Amherst, Stockbridge School of Agriculture, Amherst, Massachusetts, USA.

Jonell Sostre is a research student at Holyoke Community College, Holyoke, Massachusetts, USA.

Kazumi Tsuchiya is a doctoral student at the Center for Managing Chronic Disease, University of Michigan, Ann Arbor, Michigan, USA.

Margaret K. Wilkin is a statistician at the Center for Managing Chronic Disease, University of Michigan, Ann Arbor, Michigan, USA.

An introduction to the Food & Fitness community partnerships and this special issue

Laurie Lachance[a], Laurie Carpenter[a], Mary Emery[b] and Mia Luluquisen[c]

[a]*Center for Managing Chronic Disease, University of Michigan, Ann Arbor, USA;* [b]*ISU, NCRCRD, Ames, USA;* [c]*Alameda County Public Health Department, Office of the Director, Oakland, USA*

This special issue of *Community Development* introduces the Food and Fitness community partnerships and their work to increase access to healthy, locally grown food, and opportunities for physical activity, in vulnerable communities across the country. Established in 2007 and funded by the WK Kellogg Foundation, the partnerships are increasing the capacity of communities to participate in policy and systems change to positively affect their health and well-being. These articles together provide an illustration of how funders, grantees, and partners can work together to create sustainable change at the neighborhood level to ensure that all children and families are able to thrive.

Community-based approaches to health often focus their efforts in the many settings that influence how people think about and act in regard to health, including homes, schools, workplaces, places of worship, and other neighborhood settings (Clark et al., 2010; National Research Council, 2003a, 2003b). Lack of supportive infrastructures and broken systems in these settings make clear the importance of focusing on creating new systems that support positive health outcomes for children and families. The Food & Fitness community partnership approaches demonstrate that engaging community residents in the process of creating systems change strengthen the ability of neighborhoods, organizations, and institutions to foster and sustain those changes over time (Kubisch et al., 1997; Schulz et al., 2012).

The Food & Fitness community partnerships, funded by the W.K. Kellogg Foundation (WKKF) since 2007, were established to create community-based approaches to increase access to locally grown food and healthy places for physical activity for children and families in vulnerable communities across the United States. A critical focus of this initiative has been to create changes in policies, infrastructures, and systems that will lead not only to change, but to sustainable change. Also central to the Food & Fitness work has been the importance of engaging and empowering individuals living in these vulnerable communities so that the work derives from and is directed by the community.

The Food & Fitness community partnerships are part of a larger portfolio of investments by WKKF, known as Food & Community, which works to address some of the root causes of health inequities by transforming the food system and the built environment at local, state, regional, and national levels (WKKF, 2014). Grantees funded as part of Food & Community work to increase community access to locally grown food and opportunities for physical activity and shape the national movement toward healthy eating and active living, with the goal that all children will have an opportunity to thrive.

The Food & Fitness community partnerships

Nine culturally and geographically diverse communities in the United States were selected as Food & Fitness community partnerships to receive resources based on the readiness of agencies, organizations, institutions, and community leaders to collaborate on the development of a comprehensive plan for systems change regarding the food and active living environments. WKKF staff members were involved in suggesting and reviewing potential sites that demonstrated a readiness based on evidence of innovative programming and a history of successful collaborations. Food and Fitness communities were identified based on the following criteria: passionate leaders, especially youth leaders; involvement of critical partners like schools and churches; a network of community-based food enterprises; and past and current Foundation investments. The innovations that were already occurring in the selected communities were supported and extended with the Food & Fitness funding.

Initial funding for the partnerships provided communities with almost three years of planning support to collaboratively develop a Community Action Plan (CAP) that would guide the partnership's work. CAPs were to include methods and strategies to engage youth and community members, as well as to create cross-sector partnerships. Subsequently, partnerships received funding for five years to implement their plans.

The Boston Collaborative for Food & Fitness's (BCFF) mission has been to transform Boston, Massachusetts so that residents can access and afford healthy, locally grown food, and opportunities for active living. BCFF has focused their Food & Fitness work on neighborhoods within the city with the highest need and highest percentage of recent immigrants and the fewest opportunities for participation in the democratic process. The partnership made an early decision to work with community-based and youth organizations in these targeted neighborhoods and to allocate resources to support those organizations in their work. These conscious efforts to change practices at the neighborhood level to support increased community engagement in decision-making and the democratic process exemplify the strategic work of Food & Fitness partnerships to empower community residents.

The Detroit Food & Fitness Collaborative (DFFC) is working to remove obstacles to healthy living for children, families, and individuals living and working in this Michigan city. The collaborative includes community-based organizations, health services providers, academic institutions, youth-serving organizations, businesses, and local foundations. Operating as a catalyst in the city to create connections among organizations and individuals working in the food system and built environment, DFFC has sparked cross-sector partnerships that have effected changes across the city in expanding access to food systems and addressing challenges in the built environment.

Holyoke Food & Fitness Policy Council's (HFFPC) mission is to create and sustain a more healthy and vibrant Holyoke through the development of programs, policies, community leaders, and advocacy. Holyoke is located in the southwestern region of Massachusetts and has a population of 39,880, almost 50% of whom are Hispanic or Latino. HFFPC places an emphasis on building a community cadre of youth and community residents to better solve community issues and empower local residents to take action to improve community conditions.

The New York City Food & Fitness Partnership (NYCFAF) is an alliance whose mission is to engage communities in creating equitable access to healthy, quality, affordable foods, and opportunities for active living by working with organizations and individuals in Brooklyn, New York neighborhoods of highest need. Working to improve access to healthy food across the life span, NCYFAF is partnering with early care centers as well as farmer's markets and in the process touching upon many components of the food system.

The Northeast Iowa Food & Fitness Initiative (FFI) strives to ensure that all children and families in the six counties in their regional partnership have access to healthy, locally grown food and opportunities for physical activity. The large geographic area in which they work has necessitated a structure that integrates the work of regional and county planning teams; FFI has worked strategically to create and nurture a common vision across all of these partners, and has had great success in working with schools and local food producers to touch upon all elements in the local food chain, from production to processing, distribution, and procurement.

Health for Oakland's People and Environment Collaborative (HOPE) is working to reduce health inequalities in chronic disease related to diet and physical activity in vulnerable communities in the low-income neighborhoods of Oakland, California. HOPE strategically engages and empowers community residents with a public health approach aimed at addressing root causes of health inequalities. Their strategies are focused on creating sustainable change from the neighborhood level up by building leadership among residents most affected by health disparities while also partnering with local decision-makers, including leaders from government and for-profit businesses.

Three Food & Fitness partnerships were funded through 2013: Philadelphia Urban Food and Fitness Alliance (PUFFA), the King County Food & Fitness Initiative (KCFFI), and the Tohono O'odham Food & Fitness Collaborative. PUFFA served as a catalyst and advocate to improve access to healthy food and opportunities for physical activity in Philadelphia, Pennsylvania through connecting communities, organizations, individuals, and government, with a strong emphasis on empowering new youth leaders. An early partner of PUFFA, Common Market continues to create innovation as a mission-driven distributor of local foods to the Mid-Atlantic region. KCFFI worked to improve access to locally grown, healthy, affordable food, and safe and inviting places for physical activity and play in Delridge and White Center, two vulnerable neighborhoods in Seattle, Washington. The work of KCFFI gave rise to the very successful Food Empowerment Education and Sustainability Team (FEEST) program, a youth-led program that brings together community members to share in meals made with local food as well as conversation related to food and issues of food justice in their community. FEEST methods have been replicated in communities across the country. The Tohono O'odham Food & Fitness Collaborative, located in the Tohono O'odham nation in Pima County, Arizona, built on the community's vision of wellness by focusing on two areas: (1) capacity building, leadership development, and empowerment; and (2) creating healthy school food and fitness environments. Through their Food & Fitness funding, the collaborative was able to successfully support the creation of a new generation of farmers, focusing on culturally relevant and historic foods.

Articles in this special issue

The articles in this special issue describe many of the unique contributions of the Food & Fitness work as well as a number of early successes. They draw lessons from efforts to form and maintain partnerships, and from the strategies employed to create structural change in communities.

In the leading article, Linda Jo Doctor, Program Officer from the WKKF, sheds light on the new ways funders can operate in community-based work that allow for change emerging from community desires and needs, with funders acting in a supporting role.

The cross-site evaluation is described by the national evaluation team at the Center for Managing Chronic Disease at the University of Michigan. Born from many years of collaboration with partnerships, the cross-site evaluation underwent multiple iterations to arrive at the set of tools outlined in the article, which includes innovative measures of community-based systems and policy change.

The articles that follow from the F&F partnerships describe the structures and processes that were created to address the vision and goals of this work. To start, the work of the KCFFI created FEEST (Food Empowerment Education and Sustainability Team). The article illustrates the value placed by the WKKF on supporting youth leadership and their full participation in this work. Many of the other Food & Fitness partnerships were recipients of FEEST trainings provided by KCFFI, an example of both the opportunities for, and project leader willingness to share insights and expertise that helped create a collaboration of partners rather than a group of individual projects.

The article highlighting the work of the HOPE collaborative describes the importance of beginning with the voices of the community. HOPE began with an assessment process that engaged community members in looking at their community's strengths and opportunities, and moved into a planning and implementation process which empowered community members and youth as leaders working toward change in Oakland's food system and built environment. Authors describe the lessons learned regarding the partnership's strategic community engagement that have been gleaned from the evaluation of the partnership.

HFFPC partners share their community engagement and mobilization effort, the Call for Partnerships. The article illustrates how the strategic use of mini-grant funding can support the overall vision of the work. The authors put forth a set of strategies for utilizing mini-grant funding in ways that attract strategic partners and solidify common ground.

The Northeast Iowa FFI is a partnership that had a history of previous funding and work in the area of food systems change. FFI is an example of how the willingness of a Foundation to support work over time can reap many benefits, especially when those benefits are long-term outcomes such as policy and infrastructure changes in the food system. The article illustrating the work of FFI describes the process and outcomes of strategically aligning partners across the work, which also exemplifies the need for continual focus on common vision, even within a community with such a long history of food systems work.

The final article provides a summary of an important overarching vision for this work: closing and moving beyond the community equity gap. All of the Food & Fitness community partnerships operate in vulnerable neighborhoods and regions, and the emphasis on creating equity was explicit in the work from the outset of the initiative. The methods described in this special issue used by the partnerships to engage and empower residents move toward decreasing the equity gap; they also move beyond addressing the gap to create new structures and strategies, which are created through the introduction of a system interrupter. This final article describes such processes and illustrates how the Food & Fitness work is creating new and empowering structures that create more opportunities for health for the communities.

This initiative also created an environment to rethink how to evaluate initiative goals across geographies and strategies and in so doing developed an evaluation approach that can aid others in measuring the impact of systems change work across projects. In addition, the requirement to participate in convenings with other projects provided an opportunity for deeper learning at the project level and the broadening and deepening of networks that can help to sustain efforts into the future. Together these articles offer a view of how funders, community residents, and institutional partners can reimagine their work together in ways that address social justice concerns in the process of implementing systems change at the local and regional levels.

The Food & Fitness partnerships, funded and supported by the WKKF, bring community organizations and residents together to create healthy places where all citizens have an opportunity to engage in democratic processes and all children can thrive.

References

Clark, N. M., Lachance, L., Doctor, L. J., Gilmore, L., Kelly, C., Krieger, J., … Wilkin, M. K. (2010). Policy and system change and community coalitions: Outcomes from allies against asthma. *American Journal of Public Health, 100*, 904–912.

Kubisch, A. C., Brown, P., Chaskin, R., Hirota, J., Joseph, M., Richman, H., & Roberts, M. (1997). *Voices from the field: Learning from the early work of comprehensive community initiatives*. Washington, DC: The Aspen Institute.

National Research Council. (2003a). *The future of the public's health in the 21st century*. Washington, DC: The National Academies Press.

National Research Council. (2003b). *Who will keep the public healthy? Educating public health professionals for the 21st century*. Washington, DC: The National Academies Press.

Schulz, A. J., Mentz, G., Lachance, L., Johnson, J., Gaines, C., & Israel, B. A. (2012). Associations between socioeconomic status and allostatic load: Effects of neighborhood poverty and tests of mediating pathways. *American Journal of Public Health, 102*, 1706–1714.

W.K. Kellogg Foundation. (2014). *Food & community*. Retrieved from http://www.wkkf.org/what-we-do/healthy-kids/food-and-community

Philanthropy's role: working alongside communities to support social change

Linda Jo Doctor

W.K. Kellogg Foundation, One Michigan Avenue East, Battle Creek, USA

The field of philanthropy and funders at large can serve an important role in working alongside community to support social change. However, in doing so, the funder must answer challenging questions along the way: What is the role of a funder in supporting social and community change? How does a funder walk alongside community and support community leaders in realizing their vision? How can funders share what we learn in community with others? What can a funder do to encourage the sustainability and viability of the community programs it has helped set into motion?

In this commentary, Linda Jo Doctor, a program officer at the W.K. Kellogg Foundation, provides context and clarity around the funder's role in working alongside community partners and leaders.

Community takes the lead (funder plays a supporting role)

Philanthropic organizations have a responsibility to invest wisely, advance their mission as defined by their donor(s), and demonstrate measurable impact on the ground. This responsibility drives some to be overly prescriptive in delineating the parameters of their support, detailing their expectations, and providing specific direction about how funded work should be undertaken in community.

A different approach is for a philanthropic organization to take a step back and listen carefully to community voices, and to be receptive to ideas that emerge from a genuine and inclusive conversation among community members. The resources then follow. This is a 180° difference from a funder coming into a community and declaring: "This is what we're doing."

The W.K. Kellogg Foundation (WKKF) is fortunate to have guidance from our founder, Will Keith Kellogg, who in 1941 said, "It is only through cooperative planning, intelligent study, and group action – activities on the part of the entire community – that lasting results can be achieved." We understand this to mean that the funder follows the community as it takes the lead.

"Following" does not necessarily mean that as a funder you must remain passive or neutral. In fact, funders need to be clear from the start about their intentions and expectations; only then can the community decide whether this is the right funder for them. The funder's role is to ask questions up front, set the stage and frame the work, build connections and relationships, nurture community-driven work, share knowledge gained with the broader philanthropic field, and help the community build the capacity to sustain the work beyond the set funding period.

The experience of the Food & Fitness collaboratives raises a series of fundamental questions: What is the role of a funder in supporting social and community change? How does a funder walk alongside community and support community leaders in realizing their vision? How can funders share what we learn in community with others? What can a funder do to encourage the sustainability and viability of the community programs it has helped set into motion?

Growing hope in Oakland

In the spring of 2013, a diverse group of more than 50 residents of East Oakland, California participated in a six-session leadership academy to continue work on issues of land use, housing, transit, and food justice in their community. Among the participants were leaders from many community organizations, including Urban Habitat, Causa Justa (Just Cause), and Oakland Food Connection. The academy was sponsored by the Health for Oakland's People and Environment (HOPE) Collaborative as part of its ongoing efforts to support grassroots leaders and work with residents in the process of community transformation.

The HOPE Collaborative is one of six Food & Fitness collaboratives across the United States, part of an initiative launched in 2006 by the WKKF through its Food & Community program (Lachance, Carpenter, Emery, & Luluquisen, 2014). Each Food & Fitness collaborative works to transform food systems and the physical environment in their communities by bringing together constituencies from sustainable food systems, the built environment, economic development, and public health with youth and community residents to advance a common vision.

The collaboratives envision vibrant neighborhoods that provide equitable access to affordable, healthy, locally grown food; safe and inviting places for physical activity and play; and thriving local economies. Placing racial equity at the core of everything they do, the collaboratives believe the structural inequities that most severely impact their vulnerable communities can change only when the people living under those conditions have both civic and economic ownership of the resources and decision-making processes that impact everyday life.

Each of the Food & Fitness collaboratives began by developing a community action plan. The Kellogg Foundation provides the collaboratives with ongoing funding, along with the support and encouragement of its network of similarly engaged collaboratives. The collaboratives, in turn, draw on technical expertise, as needed, from their community partners, their peers across the country, and a set of technical assistance providers with a range of expertise. But it is the collaborative members – leadership, community partners, and residents – who developed their own vision and directed the planning. And it is collaborative members who facilitate and engage in the work of transforming their own community and determining their future.

The next two sections consider how philanthropic organizations can play this vital supporting role, drawing on the Kellogg Foundation's experience as a funder of the Food & Fitness initiative, as well as on the foundation's many decades of experience funding place-based work in the United States and internationally.

Engaging community

Architects understand that how one approaches and enters a building and how one orients to the building once inside – what some designers call the "welcoming sequence" – determines a lot about one's subsequent experience of the building. Likewise, how a funder initially enters a community sets the tone for the relationship between the funder and community partners over the course of the funding period. More importantly, it influences the relationship between the community partners and community residents and, in turn, the ultimate success and long-term viability of the funded work.

Let the community know why you're there

It may seem obvious, but before engaging a community, a philanthropic organization first must have clarity about its own purpose, goals, and reasons for funding place-based work. Upon engaging a community (regardless of whether the funder or the community partner initiated the relationship), the funder and community must be clear that they share mutual goals.

If the philanthropic organization has a particular focus or frame to its grantmaking – such as advancing equity or supporting community and civic engagement – then that focus or frame should be clearly articulated and communicated. There are many well-intentioned community-based organizations and institutions seeking funds that put forward "focus groups" or request "input" from residents and community leaders as the equity and community engagement process. For organizations providing needed services in their community, it is important to have these feedback mechanisms in place on a continuous basis as a strategy to improve their work. However, for a social change strategy that requires community, organizational, and institutional leadership, new structures need to be created and resources distributed to support ongoing engagement and participation in all aspects of the work. As the funder, it becomes imperative to ensure that all these components are in place in the beginning of the process to best reach the shared vision and goals for the work.

Acknowledge philanthropic privilege and use it well

There is an obvious power imbalance between a funder and its community partners, but it need not be an impediment to advancing work in community, so long as it is recognized by both sides.

Funders have a responsibility to leverage their access and resources to support community voice in the most authentic way possible. Philanthropic organizations must be on guard that the power and privilege inherent in their role as an outside (and often outsized) funder does not lead them to maintain inequitable structures or reinforce inequitable power dynamics in the community, thus impeding the very changes they hope to see the community make. During the initial planning phase of Food & Fitness, each of the collaboratives selected an organization to serve as the grantee on behalf of the collaborative. Early on across the sites, we saw an interesting phenomenon of "shared leadership" emerging – sometimes it was with groups across areas of content expertise, and sometimes it was across grassroots, grasstops, and institutional sectors. In every site over the course of the first five years of the project, we saw major upheavals, including changes in organizational structures and where resources were housed, many which were driven by issues of equity. As the funder, patience and flexibility are required for these organizational changes to occur, as the results of these changes only help to address complicated organizational dynamics for the better.

Community partners, in turn, need to be forthcoming about the challenges they face, as well as their triumphs, the good, and the bad in the situation on the ground. Current and potential community partners understandably want to put their best foot forward when a funder pays them a visit. What we've learned at the Kellogg Foundation through decades of investing in community is that place-based work often is messy work. In addressing structural inequities within their communities, our community partners are questioning a status quo and interrupting systems that have been in place for generations. If a community collaborative doesn't have problems or struggles, then they're perhaps not doing the work they profess to be doing. As a funder, we expect there will be challenges and want to hear about them, come to understand them, and work with our community partners to address them and move forward together.

Listen deeply

The importance of listening cannot be stressed enough. For a funder to engage a community in an authentic way requires a tremendous amount of discernment. Take a step back. You will start to understand what's happening in the community a little bit differently. Listen. You will begin to see which leaders and organizations to support. Ask questions. You will open a window on community infrastructure, both formal and informal.

Seek to understand the community on its terms. A funder cannot do this by holding focus groups or by looking through the eyes of an outside organization or agency, no matter how important a service they are providing in the community. This requires a partnership with groups on the ground that work directly with residents and that have residents in leadership positions; in other words, a partner organization that looks like the people experiencing the issues it's seeking to address.

Be inclusive

A community will thrive only when all groups and individuals have been invited to participate and feel they have a place at the table. Everyone's work is critical, so it is important to establish a viable mechanism for identifying and funding a robust mix of community voices.

In identifying who within a community to fund, philanthropic organizations should avoid gatekeepers who might close off or filter communications and access between the funder and the community. Instead, funders need to partner with organizations that have earned the trust of the community and whose connections go beneath the surface to reach not only the formal neighborhood watch group, but also the grandmother on the street who everyone knows is protecting the kids.

We felt that the participation of youth and parents was critical to the success of the Food & Fitness collaboratives, so we made a special effort to ensure that children, teens, and their parents were included in the conversation, offered a meaningful role, and supported in their growth and development as community leaders.

Work at multiple levels

A philanthropic organization can't affect change on the ground if the efforts it funds remain at the institutional level, where often large amounts of resources are required simply to support the infrastructure of the institution, and where the community voice might be muffled. Real and lasting change in community requires participation at all levels, from grassroots organizations to grasstops organizations to larger community institutions and systems. As a funder, our role has been to support the alignment of organizations working at each of these levels. In our experience, it takes at least five or six years for multi-level connections and relationships to develop, so you have to commit to funding for a long-enough period. For example, the Detroit Food & Fitness Collaborative works with organizations such as the Detroit Black Community Food Security Network; grasstops organizations such as Gleaners Community Food Bank of Southeast Michigan, Eastern Market, and Fair Food Network; and large institutions such as Detroit Public Schools. There are also new and emerging neighborhood leadership groups that have joined the collaboration, such as the Detroit Food Lab and the Osborn Neighborhood Alliance. Collaboration on all levels, from the grassroots up, has helped to foster a better alignment of resources in Detroit and has ensured that many voices continue to be heard.

Build trust and nurture authentic relationships

Above all else, in engaging in community work, a philanthropic organization must be open, honest, and transparent from the beginning. Only by establishing authentic relationships on the ground and building trust within the community can a funder hope to foster genuine partnerships that engender co-learning and lead to ongoing and enduring success.

Sustaining change

Entering and engaging a community is only the first part of a philanthropic organization's place-based work. Early on, a funder must ask: How will this work be sustained? The answer to this question – the second part of the work – involves building capacity, identifying where existing resources can be shifted, encouraging the adoption of new and innovative organizational practices, developing leaders, sharing knowledge, and helping community partners gain momentum and attract additional support and funding.

Build capacity

The role of philanthropy in building the capacity of community partners to sustain themselves continues to evolve, even as the definition of capacity building itself remains in flux. What seems clear is that lasting community change requires that the community-based organizations engaged in the work develop the capacity to improve their effectiveness and continue to fulfill their mission.

It is important that the community-based organizations themselves direct and participate fully in their own development, growth, and capacity building. Here again, philanthropic organizations can best serve communities by working alongside them.

In our work with the Food & Fitness collaboratives, the Kellogg Foundation has, by and large, fostered capacity building through technical assistance and leadership development. Much of this effort has focused on questions of power dynamics. How does a collaborative build trust between grasstops and grassroots levels, across sectors, between urban and rural constituencies, and among people addressing complex issues of race, ethnicity, and class?

We support community partners in creating a safe space for this work to take place. We also support opportunities for peer learning between the collaboratives, since with these complex subjects and issues, no one organization has all the answers. And we support technical assistance from expert advisors to address leadership development, communications capacity building, fundraising, the development of business strategies that might help sustain or generate future funding, or other expertise required for the organization to take the next steps forward.

But no matter the specific nature of the assistance, three points are critical: one, the assistance must be requested by the community partner; two, the assistance must meet a real need; and, three, the assistance must align with the partner's work and its vision for the community.

Enable community partners to learn from each other

One of the best ways to amplify efforts undertaken in community is to bring together partners from a number of communities to share with and learn from each other.

The Food & Fitness collaboratives have benefited from annual gatherings that bring together members of each collaborative to share with and learn from each other, as well as to interact with advocates, experts, and thought leaders involved in WKKF's broader Food & Community program. The gatherings are also an opportunity for community partners to deepen their understanding of issues and develop their skills in such areas as leadership, movement building, and communications.

Be patient, take your time, stay for the long haul

Philanthropic organizations must remain flexible, look constantly for creative ways to support the growth of their community partners, and be sensitive to what works for a specific community.

In particular, to do this work through the lens of racial equity, communities need time to engage in conversations, examine their own history, look at where there has been disinvestment, and understand the impact of various policies in play. It takes time to bring the people most impacted by inequities to the table and for institutional partners to align their efforts with the community's vision.

Sometimes a community partner finds its work with an institutional partner has stalled, generally around an issue of race. In cases such as this, we have served as an ally for community partners and residents to help ensure that they have a seat at the table alongside institutions.

Other times, a community partner finds that the structures it put into place at the outset need to be rebuilt. It's critical that these structures are designed from the start to be flexible and that the funder allows for structural realignment, redirection, and movement. Funding across long periods of time – five to seven years at the minimum – helps to create a flexible funding environment that allows for more reflection and realignment.

Success builds on success

What we've learned at the Kellogg Foundation is that where there is traction and progress, other funders come to the table. As philanthropic organizations, we all want to be part of something successful that can be lifted up and scaled for greater impact.

Ultimately, as a funder, you are supporting community partners to evolve their work and develop ways of sustaining it. To take its work beyond the initial funding from WKKF, one Food & Fitness collaborative, for instance, has established an endowment fund at a community foundation, along with plans to engage many local funders and ensure that future funding is equitably distributed. The idea is that, over time, community partners and institutions change their organizational practices and realign their own resources to continue the work. This is how community-driven change is sustained.

It takes courage to work differently.

Reference

Lachance, L., Carpenter, L., Emery, M., & Luluquisen, M. (2014). An introduction to the Food & Fitness community partnerships and this special issue. *Community Development*. 45: 3, 215–219.

Food & Community: the cross-site evaluation of the W.K. Kellogg Food & Fitness community partnerships

Laurie Lachance[a], Laurie Carpenter[a], Martha Quinn[a], Margaret K. Wilkin[a], Edward Green[a], Kazumi Tsuchiya[a], Belinda Nelson[a], Cleopatra Caldwell[a], Linda Jo Doctor[b] and Noreen M. Clark[a]

[a]*Center for Managing Chronic Disease, University of Michigan, USA;*
[b]*W.K. Kellogg Foundation, East Battle Creek, USA*

This article describes the collaborative development of the cross-site evaluation of the Food & Fitness initiative. Evaluators and community partners together created a multi-site evaluation to document similarities and unique aspects across the work in the nine participating communities. The evaluation includes measures of partner engagement, resources, processes, and outcomes of achieving systems and policy change, and impact of the work in vulnerable communities. Inherent in and critical to the evaluation is a process for providing feedback to communities and stakeholders. Pioneering ways to assess the process of achieving systems and policy change and the impact of this work on children and families, the Food & Fitness cross-site evaluation is creating a picture of the collective accomplishments of these community partnerships, which are doing innovative work related to equity around food access and the built environment.

Differences in the opportunities for health promoting services and activities across neighborhoods in the US influence lifestyle behaviors critical to maintaining health and preventing chronic disease (Larson, Story, & Nelson, 2009; Lovasi, Hutson, Guerra, & Neckerman, 2009). Lack of opportunity has been linked to inequities evident in low-income communities. Individual behavior is acknowledged as shaped by systemic, avoidable, unjust, community-wide disparities in access that in turn affect health status and the distribution of morbidity and mortality across neighborhoods (Epping-Jordan, Pruitt, Bengoa, & Wagner, 2004; Frieden, Dietz, & Collins, 2010; Schmid, Pratt, & Howze, 1995; Story, Kaphingst, Robinson-O'Brien, & Glanz, 2008). Health improvement has been seen as dependent on decreasing the equity gap (Clark et al., 2011; Israel et al., 2010; Livingood et al., 2011). Equity in this regard refers to assumptions, practices, and institutional behaviors that reform the social structures that consistently consign too few benefits and too many obstacles for health to those in vulnerable neighborhoods, especially poor people of color (Institute for Democratic Renewal and Project Change Anti-Racism Initiative, 2001).

Efforts to increase health equity are influenced by the complex social and physical environments where vulnerable families and children live, work, and play. Availability of healthy food and safe places for physical activity is less evident in low-income neighborhoods, and particularly low-income neighborhoods of color (Auchincloss et al., 2009; Franco, Diez Roux, Glass, Caballero, & Brancati, 2008; Landrine & Corral, 2009). Numerous studies have identified targeted policy change as a promising strategy for creating infrastructure, services, and activities that can yield population-wide improvements in diet, physical activity, and prevalence of obesity-related conditions (Brownson, Haire-Joshu, & Luke, 2006; Frieden et al., 2010; Papas et al., 2007; Sacks, Swinburn, & Lawrence, 2009).

Community-based approaches provide opportunities to influence the complex social and physical environments that shape opportunities for health by strengthening the ability of neighborhood residents, organizations, and institutions to foster and sustain neighborhood change (DeFilippis, 2001; Kubisch, Auspos, Brown, & Dewar, 2010; Schulz et al., 2013). Building capacity within communities towards change is a democratic process that provides residents with the tools to be agents of their own change, rather than beneficiaries of change, creating opportunities for community members to be included in discussions and decisions about what should be done and how change efforts should be accomplished (Clark et al., 2006). Efforts that involve community members underscore the values of equity, self-determination, social justice, and respect for diversity that are fundamental to healthy communities (Clark et al., 2006; DeFilippis, 2001; Kubisch et al., 2010)

Through Food & Community – a program of the W.K. Kellogg Foundation (WKKF) – national, regional, and local partners are working to effect policy and system change that will transform school food systems, community access to good food and physical activity, and contribute to the national movement for healthy eating and active living (Lachance, Carpenter, Emery, & Luluquisen, 2014). This work aims to address inequities and the root causes of poor health so that all children have the opportunity to thrive. As part of Food & Community, the Food & Fitness community partnerships were formed in 2007. The intention was to create vibrant, healthy environments in selected vulnerable neighborhoods across the US. Children, youth, and families would be helped by making available and promoting consumption of healthy food, and through the creation of safe spaces and infrastructures for physical activity, that is increased opportunities for developing healthy behaviors and enhancing overall health and well-being. The Food & Fitness partnerships comprise community-based, local collaborations engaged in targeted change efforts, and share the vision and purpose of the WKKF's overarching Food & Community Program.

Partners are diverse and include individuals and representatives of organizations focused on changing food systems and the built environment in communities and schools. The food systems change partners represent all elements of the food production, processing, distribution, and retail segments, and include farmers, food distributors, food processors, food service directors, farmer's market staff, and food retailers. All segments of schools and community are represented, including city planners, transportation and housing authority, parks and recreation departments, health departments, community and economic development organizations, mayoral staff, school boards, school principals, teachers, parents, and students. Civic engagement and capacity building are emphasized within the partnerships, along with creating opportunities for diverse leadership. Particular efforts are made to build the capacity of youth, both within schools and the overall community. Technical assistance to the partners is provided through a wide range of consultants within and outside of the WKKF. Assistance emphasizes both content (food systems, school food change, active living, built environment) and process (policy change, partnership facilitation, visioning) of the work.

From the start, there was an emphasis in the work of the community partnerships to ensure the sustainability of changes realized. To this end, Food & Fitness partnerships have created a process for identifying change opportunities, prioritizing change efforts, and building capacity for contributing to local policy and systems change. Civic and youth engagement have been a focus and means to develop leaders who can influence and become decision-makers. Many targeted local changes of the Food & Fitness community partnerships link to policy goals at the regional, state, tribal, and national levels and reflect the focus of other WKKF investments.

The Food & Fitness community partnerships, by design, bring multiple sectors together to garner critical perspectives and resources and to mobilize stakeholders toward common goals. The aim is to develop asset-based solutions that foster empowerment, self-determination, and resilience. These partnerships have been deliberate in their efforts to achieve health equity in two ways: first, by focusing on neighborhoods where divestment has been occurring over many years, in most cases because of structural racism; and second, by focusing efforts in communities where partnerships already existed and comprised the foundation for greater civic engagement and inclusion of often unheard community voices in decisions regarding community change.

Communities in nine areas were chosen to begin the Food & Fitness partnership work: Boston, Detroit, Holyoke, Northeast Iowa, New York City, Oakland, Philadelphia, Seattle/King County, and the Tohono O'odham Nation. Evaluation was embedded within and across these partnerships from the start. Partners and a national cross-site evaluation team collaboratively designed the evaluation methods and tools and implemented data collection in concert. As part of the process, representatives from the nine partnerships, including the local evaluators, came together initially with a scientific evaluation advisory group to discuss potential measures of change efforts applicable across the communities. Challenges from the beginning included the need to demonstrate both outcomes and an understanding of how the outcomes occurred. Another challenge related to the latter processes is how to describe the partnership and ways members worked together to create change. Although some partners had worked together for decades, shifting their efforts away from programs and services toward policy and infrastructure change created new challenges for many. A different type of partnering was needed to effect long-term impact vs. provision of short-term programs. The design of the cross-site evaluation needed to capture elements of partnership over time in relation to accomplishments and challenges, processes, and outcomes.

Design of the cross-site evaluation

It was part of the WKKF vision for the Food & Fitness initiative to explore common goals across the nine partnerships and create common methods for the most important elements of the evaluation. The overall approach of the Food & Fitness cross-site evaluation was to use a collaborative process to document similarities and unique aspects of the work in nine participating communities. The cross-site tools were the means to track the involvement of partners engaged in the work, resources brought into the partnership, the systems and policy change process undertaken, outcomes achieved, and the impact of those outcomes on children and families in vulnerable neighborhoods. Assessments of civic and youth engagement, capacity building, and a focus on equity were incorporated throughout the evaluation methods and tools because, as noted, they represent core values of the Food & Fitness community partnerships.

Development of the cross-site evaluation tools was a critical task over the two-year planning phase (2007–2008) of the Food & Fitness initiative (see Figure 1). As an initial step, an evaluation advisory group was formed of national experts to oversee the design and ensure that the evaluation would focus on addressing equity. Several face-to-face meetings took place with representatives of the partners, including local evaluators and the University of Michigan Center for Managing Chronic Disease (UM-CMCD) cross-site evaluation team, to exchange ideas and work out the details of the cross-site evaluation.

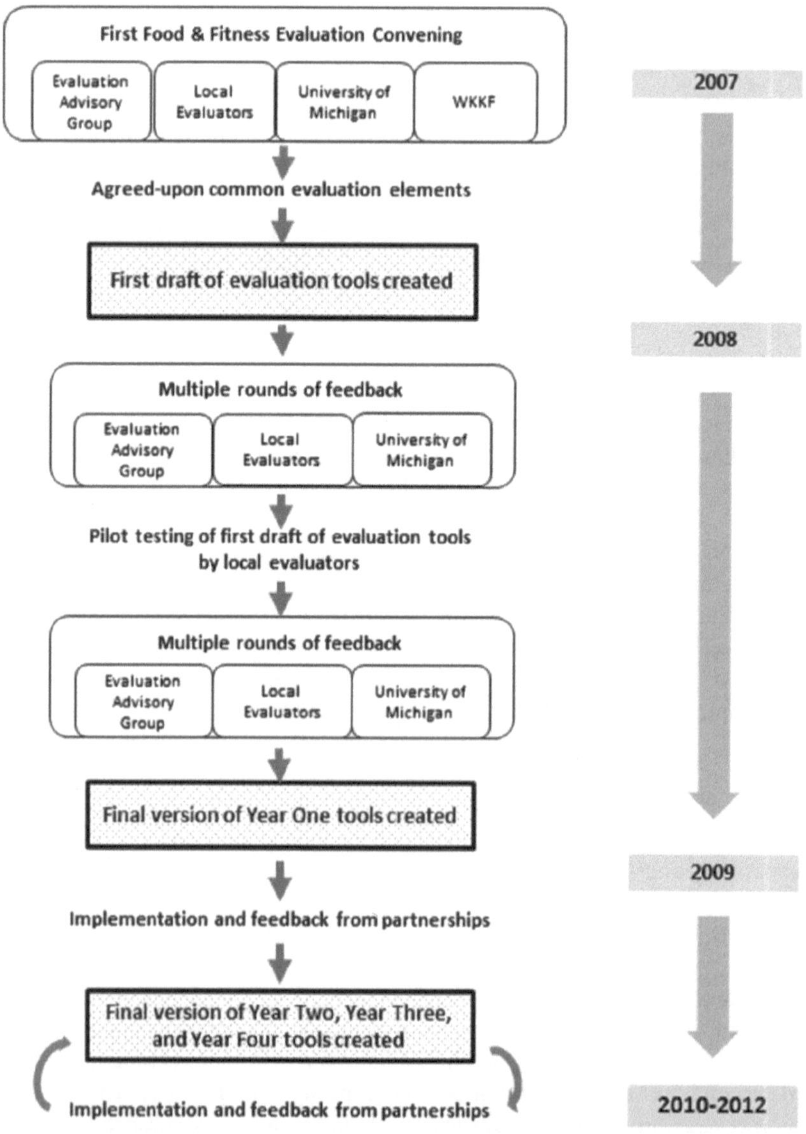

Figure 1. Development of the Food & Fitness Cross-Site Evaluation.

During the first Food & Fitness evaluation meeting in July 2007, the local evaluators, the UM-CMCD evaluation team, and the Evaluation Advisory Group worked together to create the foundation of the Food & Fitness cross-site evaluation. At a subsequent meeting in October 2007, the objectives and measures were further honed, and the first version of the cross-site tools emerged from that meeting. To ensure the credibility of the tools, input was requested from content area experts as well as other Food & Fitness, technical assistance providers.

After initial revisions based on this feedback, the first draft of the cross-site evaluation tools was sent to the local community evaluators for their feedback in January 2008. All communities provided feedback to the UM team regarding this initial draft. This feedback led to a number of changes to the tools: adding items sensitive to particular cultures and settings, removing items deemed too burdensome to be included in the data collection after weighing the benefits of collection with the resources needed, adding items considered helpful to the work of the partnerships, clarifying items, and modifying the methods for data collection and reporting.

A second version of the cross-site evaluation tools was developed based on the comprehensive input provided by the partnerships and the Evaluation Advisory Group. The revised set of tools was sent to the partnerships for feedback in June 2008, and was also discussed at length during the Evaluation Advisory Group Meeting that same month. Again, each local evaluation team provided feedback regarding the second version of the proposed cross-site evaluation tools.

Based on the feedback received from both the communities and the Evaluation Advisory Group on the second iteration of the cross-site evaluation tools, Version 3 was developed. Examples of changes made based on feedback received include a stronger emphasis on youth partners in the Collaborative Partners Form, additional details added to the Systems and Policy Change Stories, and a number of additions to the Systems and Policy Change Form to reflect more of the process of systems and policy change, in addition to the outcomes.

The third version of the cross-site evaluation tools was shared with the local evaluation teams prior to the evaluation meeting in February 2009, and feedback was given to the UM team during conference calls with evaluators and other members of the partnerships. This feedback led to the development of the fourth iteration of the tools, which were shared during the February 2009 evaluation meeting with the local evaluators and the Evaluation Advisory Group. Also shared during this meeting was information collected from further pilot testing of the tools by the local evaluation teams. Over the spring of 2009, modifications were made to the tools based on discussions that took place during the February evaluation meeting and the further pilot testing by the local evaluators.

To ensure the effectiveness and efficiency of the tools, all components were pilot tested by the local evaluation teams using participatory methods. The Health for Oakland's People and Environment (HOPE) Collaborative pilot tested the *Collaborative Partners* tool, the Northeast Iowa Food & Fitness Initiative pilot tested the *Resource Tracking* tool, the Philadelphia Urban Food & Fitness Alliance (PUFFA) pilot tested the *Systems and Policy Change Stories* tool, and the Detroit Food & Fitness Collaborative piloted the *Systems and Policy Change* tracking tool. Results from the final pilot testing were used to refine the tools and to provide example methods for participatory approaches to data collection that other partnerships could employ. Examples of these approaches that arose from the pilot testing include: meeting with partnership work groups, leadership, and staff to gather information about partners, change efforts, resources, and efforts to track through stories; reviewing secondary data (budgets, media pieces, and memorandums of understanding [MOUs]) for information about ongoing efforts; and interviewing community partners involved in the work.

At the conclusion of the spring of 2009, all tools that comprised the cross-site evaluation were pilot tested and vetted by the local Food & Fitness evaluation teams.

The cross-site tools were finalized, and baseline data were collected in November 2009; annual data collection is ongoing. All partnerships use participatory methods to collect data that include local evaluators working with partnership leaders and other stakeholders to gain multiple perspectives on the partnership, processes, outcomes, and impact of the work using the cross-site evaluation tools to document and track changes. Further information about the methods used for these tools is described in more detail below.

Cross-site evaluation tools

The Food & Fitness cross-site evaluation tools tap three elements of the community partnerships' work: (1) collaborative partnerships; (2) resource acquisition; and (3) systems and policy change.

Four tools yield quantitative and qualitative information on these elements that can be used cross-sectionally and longitudinally to understand the changes that occur in each community. The tools are available at the website of the Center for Managing Chronic Disease at the University of Michigan (http://managingchronicdisease.org).

Details about each cross-site evaluation tool are summarized below, followed by methods used to collect and track data over time, additional sources of data for the cross-site evaluation, and how evaluation data are used for decision-making.

Collaborative Partners

The objective of the *Collaborative Partners Form* tool is to document and track individual and organizational partners comprising the community partnership, and the level of diversity in engagement and multi-sector collaboration. The tool guides local evaluation teams to report five types of partners: (1) *core individual and organizational partners* – people and organizations central to the functioning of the partnership, decision-makers for major actions of the partnership; (2) *ongoing individual and organizational partners* – people and/or organizations who are not as central to the partnership's functioning as the core partners but are often present, important to the ongoing effort, and make regular contributions; (3) *strategic individual and organizational partners* – individuals and organizations that the partnership turns to for added help at strategic times with systems and policy change work, not present often, but are important for realizing particular objectives; (4) *targeted potential allies beyond the partnership* – those in the wider environment beyond the partnership who are not involved, and needed to achieve the targeted systems and policy changes; and (5) *potential challengers* – people/organizations who are not partners, and may be in opposition to the partnership's efforts.

The *Collaborative Partners* tool is used to track the type of group, organization, or entity the representative member is affiliated with (i.e. community-based organization, community-based agency, non-profit, for-profit, government, school, academic/research institution, individual, and other). Information is tracked regarding the primary focus and nature of the individual's work in the partnership (i.e. food production, food processing, food distribution, institutional food service, food retail, physical activity, built environment, health, youth development, community development, economic development, civic engagement, schools, and other). Roles in the partnership are tracked over the duration of the work (2008–Present), and the tool provides an opportunity to identify responsibilities (i.e. convener, fiduciary agent, project director/program coordinator, evaluator, other project staff, steering/executive committee chair, steering/executive committee member, other committee/work group chair, other committee/work group member, adult member – not part of any committee or work group, youth member – not part of any committee or work group, and other). For each participant, information is collected about the specific systems and policy change efforts in which the individual or organization is engaged and whether the representative is a youth or adult partner. The classification of partners can be analyzed cross-sectionally and longitudinally, within and across the nine partnerships, to describe the patterns of participation, and to ascertain any correlations these patterns may have with outcomes of interest in the initiative.

Resource tracking

Major resources that are brought into and leveraged by the partnerships are tracked using the *Resource Tracking Form* tool. Documentation of the resources includes the type of resource (i.e. money, full-time equivalent of work), the source, and the specific work of the partnership that the resource will support. These data enable description of the magnitude of resources and how they are deployed by the partnerships. In this form, partnerships are instructed to verify and document the resource acquired or the commitment made (e.g. a budget line or notation, MOU, or a letter stating intent). In addition to documenting the resources obtained by the partnerships, there is an option to track resources aligned with the systems and policy change targets of the partnership. Aligned resources are those that support similar goals in the community to those of the Food & Fitness partnerships, but do not directly support the work of the partnership. Some examples of reported aligned resources include CDC grants that support expansion of community gardens, USDA funding to support farmers and farmers' markets, and city funds to improve community parks. In several cases, members of the partnerships played a role in securing these funds, from garnering community support to participating on committees.

Tracking the flow of resources can illustrate the increased acquisition and leveraging of resources in the form of matching funds, in-kind support, and additional grants and contracts to further the partnerships' work over time.

Systems and policy change

Systems and policy changes are documented in two ways: process and outcome tracking of specific efforts, and stories.

Systems and policy change tracking

Systems and policy changes that result from efforts in which the partnerships provide leadership or make a critical contribution to the effort are documented over the length of the project through the use of a comprehensive tracking tool, the *Systems and Policy Change Form* tool.

Indicators regarding both process and outcome data are collected with this tool, including the estimated or measured impact on the community. The tool also tracks strategies, tactics, and linkages formed to achieve change. The tool collects information regarding perceptions of those involved regarding how the proposed changes address equity and how they will have an impact on children and families in vulnerable communities (i.e. improved access to affordable, healthy food, and safe places to be physically active and play).

Influence of the partnership in the change efforts is categorized as: leader of the effort; shared leadership with other groups; or contributing collaborator, that is lending support. The phase of change is reported as: *beginning*, where the partnership has identified and agreed upon goals, strategies have been developed, strategic partners have been formed, and support and momentum for change are growing; *proposed plan drafted or introduced*, where the partnership has drafted, introduced, or submitted proposed changes to a governing authority, which are being considered by the decision-making body (this stage can include an application for funding, or revisions in proposed changes); *adoption*, where the change has been adopted by the decision-making body and documented in memos, guidelines, regulations, or laws (this stage might also include elimination of a policy or regulation); *implementation*, where there is evidence of action towards the change, including budget appropriations and other evidence of built capacity; or *maintenance/enforcement*, where efforts are underway to ensure that the change and funding for the change is available and accessed, and that a system for monitoring the policy over time has been established.

Because the efforts of the Food & Fitness community partnerships focus on increasing equity, the tool captures information about how the change will address equity, specifically how it will increase access (including affordability) to healthy, locally grown food and safe places for physical activity for children and families in the community who are most burdened or traditionally overlooked. Another aspect of equity assessed is increased capacity in the community to include the voices of conventionally unheard residents.

Stories

The *Systems and Policy Change Stories* tool gives partnerships the opportunity to showcase efforts toward change they deem compelling as they consider their efforts in given time windows. Stories convey history, identity, and culture through descriptive narrative. The stories tool asks partnerships to provide descriptions in narrative form of two change efforts per year. The tool includes suggested story protocols that ask for details regarding the specific objectives, setting, partners, resources involved, outcomes, impact on the community, lessons learned, and other pertinent elements that help provide a qualitative picture of the process of moving toward systems and policy change. This provides an opportunity for describing elements of the partnerships' efforts including, (a) a process of full engagement of community partners and diverse voices in the pursuit of change, (b) an increasing ability to overcome barriers to systems and policy change, and (c) evidence of efforts and/or examples of development of new economic endeavors associated with the partnerships' work. The stories submitted by the partnerships provide a richness of detail that can inform how outcomes emerge.

Methods

The local evaluator is responsible for reporting the data using the cross-site tools to UM-CMCD and WKKF on an annual basis. Although methods for collecting data are developed within each partnership and reported along with the data, all partnerships use comparable methods that include tracking information on an ongoing basis; consulting with the partnership leadership, partners, and other stakeholders; and providing multiple opportunities for partnership members to contribute information and respond to data being reported. These methods were collaboratively developed and shared across the partnerships during the pilot phase of the cross-site tool design, and guide the process for the cross-site evaluation.

Critical elements of the participatory methods used by the partnerships include:

- Meet with the local working groups, action teams, and committees to collaboratively complete tools related to their specific work.
- Determine with project leadership the most efficacious ways to track efforts according to the three main areas of the work (i.e. school food, community food, and active living/built environment).
- Interview community partners and other stakeholders involved in the efforts in order to gain multiple perspectives on the issues and to include a rich collection of details in the tracking and stories (e.g. school food directors, local decision makers, and public health department officials).
- Collect primary data in targeted communities collaboratively with youth, community partners, and project staff (e.g. farmers' markets surveys, observation of built environment usage, interviews with community members, and surveys of food availability).
- Review secondary data (e.g. budgets, MOUs, partnership meeting minutes, media outlets, and documents from organizational partners).
- Meet regularly with all members of the evaluation team to address any duplications or inconsistencies.

Once tools are submitted, the UM-CMCD team goes through an initial verification process to make sure information is complete. The UM-CMCD team then follows up with each local evaluator individually to make the necessary changes to the data. This may involve several conversations that include partnership leaders and stakeholders.

Additional sources of data for the cross-site evaluation

Several sources of information are utilized in addition to the data collected by the partnerships using the cross-site evaluation tools. They include the WKKF grantee annual reports and key informant interviews with the partnership leadership and staff, in addition to community partners and youth members.

The annual report to WKKF allows evaluators, project directors, and staff to document the processes, structures, and outcomes of the work of the partnership, using the requisite guidelines distributed annually by WKKF. Project directors and local evaluators work together and with the partnership leadership to determine how the annual report is completed. Project directors are responsible for reporting the information annually to WKKF.

The key informant interviews commenced during the planning phase and continue on a regular basis. To date, three sets of interviews have been completed between 2008 and 2012 ($n = 82$, 86 and 101, respectively). The fourth set of interviews is currently underway. An average of 9–11 participants from each partnership are referred for interview by the project directors. Informants are followed for subsequent years, unless they leave the partnership. The interview protocol includes a series of open-ended questions about the informants' perspectives on the partnership's greatest accomplishments, challenges, and surprises; the lessons they have learned about community and youth engagement; and their views on how the work of the partnership is increasing equity in their community. All interviews are conducted on the telephone, recorded, transcribed, and analyzed to understand common themes that emerge across all partnerships, as well as themes that are unique to individual partnerships. All of the elements of the Food & Fitness cross-site evaluation, including roles and responsibilities for reporting of the data, are listed in Table 1.

Evaluation feedback

A large cross-site evaluation holds potential for generating data regarding the collective effort and findings for individual partnerships. An important consideration is how information regarding processes and outcomes can be shared with stakeholders in an ongoing way to contribute to refinements and anticipate challenges in the work. In keeping with principles of community-based participatory research (Israel et al., 2001; Schulz, Israel, Selig, Bayer, & Griffin, 1998), feedback and integration of evaluation results are critical to the ongoing work. The Food & Fitness Cross-Site Evaluation has introduced the idea of creating a feedback loop for evaluation (see Figure 2). After the local evaluation teams report data, the UM-CMCD team provides analyses describing the multi-site venture to all partnerships and data to each individual partnership regarding their specific efforts. Partnership leaders are encouraged to share ongoing findings with their partners and members and determine their own best way to do this. Examples include sharing findings regarding partnership engagement with working groups in order to make decisions about which partners are not involved but may be helpful to engage in order to achieve partnership goals, and reviewing outcomes with the partnership steering

Table 1. Elements of the cross-site evaluation: Food & Fitness community partnerships.

Measure	Tool	Responsible party
Measures of collaboration and youth and community engagement over time	Collaborative Partners Form	Local evaluators
Tracking of resources brought into and leveraged by the partnerships and aligned resources in the community	Resource Tracking Form	Local evaluators
Documentation of context, processes, and structure involved in achieving systems and policy changes	Systems and Policy Change Stories	Local evaluators
Documentation of systems and policy changes, outcomes, and impact on vulnerable children and families	Systems and Policy Change Form	Local evaluators
Documentation of processes, structure, and work of the partnerships	Annual Report	Project directors/staff
Documentation of lessons learned by the partnership leaders and staff, youth members, and community members working with the partnerships	Lessons Learned Interviews	UM evaluation team

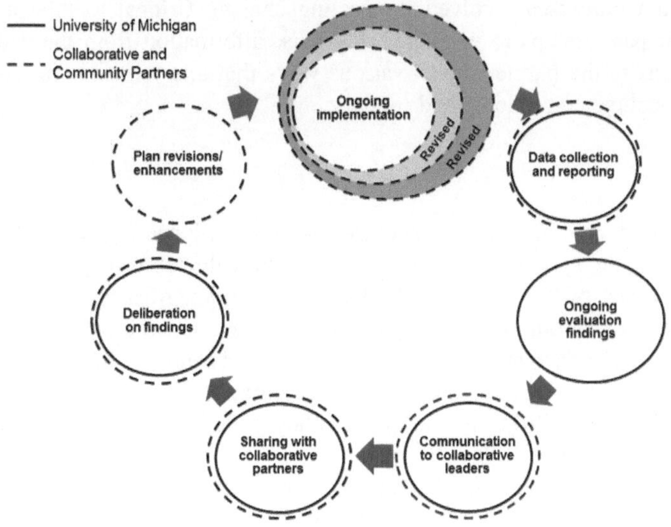

Figure 2. Food & Fitness evaluation feedback loop.

committee during the process of revising the partnership objectives. The aim is to enable partnerships to fine tune and focus their efforts.

The parallel objectives of the feedback loop are to:

(1) *Inform ongoing partnership work at the local level.* Pulling data from the cross-site tools enables shared lessons learned, and documentation of movement towards overall goals and outcomes. They provide the basis for partners individually and collectively, within and across partnerships, to participate in ongoing discussions and interpretation of findings, help verify the evaluation process, and also enrich the dialog within the partnerships for deciding how to do their work.

(2) *Inform the field.* The multi-site evaluation has great potential for informing others working toward sustainable changes in their community food, school food, active living, and built environment. Cross-site data can provide both quantitative and qualitative results related to types of changes, and how those changes are occurring. Analyses in the Food & Fitness Cross-Site Evaluation focus particularly on how changes influence the development of civic engagement, self-determined efforts that build local economic structures, and evidence of sustainable changes. Food & Fitness community partnerships are being viewed by others as experts and models in this type of work, and findings will inform not only practitioners but also the literature, funders, and other stakeholders.

A continual feedback process has been in place and continues to operate throughout the implementation of the cross-site evaluation. Monthly telephone calls, on-site meetings, and convening at the national gatherings provide opportunities for feedback to occur both from the UM team to the partnerships, and from the partnerships back to the team. This feedback loop includes opportunities for partnership members and technical assistance providers to participate in discussions related to documentation and reporting of successes and processes involved in creating change. Critical to this process is the opportunity for partnerships to use and bring back information from the evaluation and these discussions to the partnership in various ways that allow for ongoing reflection on the work, mid-course corrections, and innovation.

Conclusion

The WKKF Food & Fitness cross-site evaluation is pioneering ways to assess the process of achieving systems and policy change in vulnerable neighborhood environments and the effect of this work on children and families. Measures of the evaluation, including partner collaboration, leveraging of resources, and the process and outcomes of systems and policy change efforts, together create a picture of the innovative community-based work being done by the community partnerships. Aggregating data across the nine communities allows for in-depth analyses of similarities, differences, and collective accomplishments.

Efforts to capture information related to community change require inclusion of multiple stakeholders having ongoing opportunities for contributing to the documentation related to the process and outcomes of the work. Best results are obtained when multiple voices are included in the evaluation, and when partnership-specific work is tracked in an ongoing manner with regular opportunities for collaborative feedback and reflection. Evaluation feedback is critical to the continued development and improvement of both the work and the evaluation, and valuable to others doing similar work in the community.

As the Food & Fitness community partnerships have emerged as exemplary efforts working to increase community capacity to change neighborhood food and physical activity environments, cross-site evaluation data are critical to document and share experiences and outcomes.

Acknowledgements

We gratefully acknowledge the guidance and contributions of the evaluation advisory group: Ross C. Brownson, Cleopatra H. Caldwell, Eugenia (Geni) Eng, Robert (Bob) M. Goodman, Michael Hamm, Sherman James, Bobby Milstein, Gayle Peterson, and John Sherman; evaluators from the community partnerships: Chris Navin and Marian Milbauer (Navin Associates), Catherine Sands and Carol Stewart (Partnership in Practice), Jane Morgan (JFM Consulting Group, Inc.), Allen Cheadle, Bill Beery, Ron Maynard, Madeleine Frey, Diana Charbonneau (Group Health Research Institute), Corry Bregendahl (Leopold Center for Sustainable Agriculture), Pam Koch, Heewon Lee, and Isobel Contento (Teachers College at Columbia University), Cornelia Flora (North Central Regional Center for Rural Development at Iowa State University), Mary Emery (Iowa State University), Mia Luluquisen, Anaa Reese, and Lauren Pettis (Alameda County Public Health Department), Rickie Brawer (Thomas Jefferson University and Hospital), Kathleen Coughey (Public Health Management Corporation), Susan Lobo, and Paul Buseck; the dedicated members of all of the Food & Fitness community partnerships; and the ongoing support of the W.K. Kellogg Foundation.

References

Auchincloss, A. H., Roux, A. V. D., Mujahid, M. S., Shen, M., Bertoni, A. G., & Carnethon, M. R. (2009). Neighborhood resources for physical activity and healthy foods and incidence of type 2 diabetes mellitus: The multiethnic study of atherosclerosis. *Archives of Internal Medicine, 169*, 1698–1704.

Brownson, R. C., Haire-Joshu, D., & Luke, D. A. (2006). Shaping the context of health: A review of environmental and policy approaches in the prevention of chronic diseases. *Annual Review of Public Health, 27*, 341–370.

Clark, N. M., Brenner, J., Johnson, P., Peek, M., Spoonhunter, H., Walton, J., … Nelson, B. (2011). Reducing disparities in diabetes: The alliance model for health care improvements. *Diabetes Spectrum, 24*, 226–230.

Clark, N. M., Doctor, L. J., Friedman, A. R., Lachance, L. L., Houle, C. R., Geng, X. & Grisso, J. A. (2006). Community coalitions to control chronic disease: Allies against asthma as a model and case study. *Health Promotion Practice, 7*, 14S–22S.

DeFilippis, J. (2001). The myth of social capital in community development. *Housing Policy Debate, 12*, 781–806.

Epping-Jordan, J. E., Pruitt, S. D., Bengoa, R., & Wagner, E. H. (2004). Improving the quality of health care for chronic conditions. *Quality and Safety in Health Care, 13*, 299–305.

Franco, M., Diez Roux, A. V., Glass, T. A., Caballero, B., & Brancati, F. L. (2008). Neighborhood characteristics and availability of healthy foods in Baltimore. *American Journal of Preventive Medicine, 35*, 561–567.

Frieden, T. R., Dietz, W., & Collins, J. (2010). Reducing childhood obesity through policy change: Acting now to prevent obesity. *Health Affairs, 29*, 357–363.

Institute for Democratic Renewal and Project Change Anti-Racism Initiative. (2001). *A community builder's tool kit: 15 tools for creating healthy, productive interracial/multicultural communities*. Claremont, CA: Claremont Graduate University.

Israel, B. A., Coombe, C. M., Cheezum, R. R., Schulz, A. J., McGranaghan, R. J., Lichtenstein, R., … Akosua, B. (2010). Community-based participatory research: A capacity-building approach for policy advocacy aimed at eliminating health disparities. *American Journal of Public Health, 100*, 2094–2102.

Israel, B. A., Lichtenstein, R., Lantz, P., McGranaghan, R., Allen, A., Guzman, R. J., Softley, D., & Maciak, B. (2001). The Detroit Community-Academic Urban Research Center: Development, implementation, and evaluation. *Journal of Public Health Management and Practice, 7*, 1–19.

Kubisch, A. C., Auspos, P., Brown, P., & Dewar, T. (2010). *Voices from the field III: Lessons and challenges from two decades of community change efforts*. Washington, DC: Aspen Institute.

Lachance, L., Carpenter, L., Emery, M., & Luluquisen, M. (2014). An introduction to the Food & Fitness community partnerships and this special issue. *Community Development, 45*, 215–219.

Landrine, H., & Corral, I. (2009). Separate and unequal: Residential segregation and black health disparities. *Ethnicity & Disease, 19*, 179–184.

Larson, N. I., Story, M. T., & Nelson, M. C. (2009). Neighborhood environments: Disparities in access to healthy foods in the U.S. *American Journal of Preventive Medicine, 36*, 74–81.

Livingood, W. C., Allegrante, J. P., Airhihenbuwa, C. O., Clark, N. M., Windsor, R. C., Zimmerman, M. A., & Green, L. W. (2011). Applied social and behavioral science to address complex health problems. *American Journal of Preventive Medicine, 41*, 525–531.

Lovasi, G. S., Hutson, M. A., Guerra, M., & Neckerman, K. M. (2009). Built environments and obesity in disadvantaged populations. *Epidemiologic Reviews, 31*, 7–20.

Papas, M. A., Alberg, A. J., Ewing, R., Helzlsouer, K. J., Gary, T. L., & Klassen, A. C. (2007). The built environment and obesity. *Epidemiologic Reviews, 29*, 129–143.

Sacks, G., Swinburn, B., & Lawrence, M. (2009). Obesity policy action framework and analysis grids for a comprehensive policy approach to reducing obesity. *Obesity reviews, 10*, 76–86.

Schmid, T. L., Pratt, M., & Howze, E. (1995). Policy as intervention: Environmental and policy approaches to the prevention of cardiovascular disease. *American Journal of Public Health, 85*, 1207–1211.

Schulz, A. J., Israel, B. A., Selig, S. M., Bayer, I. S., & Griffin, C. B. (1998). Development and implementation of principles for community-based research in public health. In R. H. MacNair (Ed.), *Research strategies for community practice* (pp. 83–110). New York, NY: Haworth Press.

Schulz, A. J., Mentz, G., Lachance, L. L., Zenk, S. N., Johnson, J., Stokes, C., & Mandell, R. (2013). Do observed or perceived characteristics of the neighborhood environment mediate associations between neighborhood poverty and cumulative biological risk? *Health & Place, 24*, 147–156.

Story, M., Kaphingst, K. M., Robinson-O'Brien, R., & Glanz, K. (2008). Creating healthy food and eating environments: Policy and environmental approaches. *Annual Review of Public Health, 29*, 253–272.

FEEST on this: youth engagement for community change in the King County Food and Fitness Initiative

Diana Rowland Charbonneau[a], Allen Cheadle[a], Cristina Orbé[b], Madeline Frey[c] and Brad Gaolach[d]

[a]*Group Health Research Institute, Center for Community Health & Evaluation, USA;* [b]*WCCDA, FEEST, USA;* [c]*Healthcare Georgia Foundation, Atlanta, USA;* [d]*Washington State University Extension, Extension Community and Economic Development Program Unit, Tacoma, USA*

Empowering youth to affect change in their lives and their communities can result in healthier youth and communities. The Food Empowerment Education and Sustainability Team (FEEST) engages youth 12–24 in two ethnically diverse communities in King County, WA around food justice and food systems. At FEEST, youth and adults participate as equals. The core of the program is weekly dinners where youth cook and eat local fresh food while engaging in facilitated discussions about community, local food systems, and the role social determinants of health play in access to healthy food. A second core component is the paid youth internship program. Since FEEST's inception in 2008 through 2012, there have been over 900 participants in dinners and over 36 paid interns. Key success factors include: egalitarian youth–adult relationships, youth-driven programming, clear roles and expectations, project-based learning with paid internships, and using food and community meals as the convening platform.

Background

Healthy eating impacts the lives of the youth in this country; it helps prevent high cholesterol and high blood pressure and helps reduce the risk of developing chronic diseases such as cardiovascular disease, cancer, and diabetes (Dietary Guidelines Advisory Committee, 2010). However, many of our youth are not eating healthily. Over the past 30 years, childhood obesity rates in America have more than tripled, reaching epidemic levels: today, nearly one in three children in America is overweight or obese (Centers for Disease Control and Prevention, 2012). Children and adolescents who are obese are likely to become obese as adults (Freedman et al., 2005, 2009; Freedman, Kahn, Dietz, Srinivasan, & Berenson, 2001; Guo & Chumlea, 1999; Whitaker, Wright, Pepe, Seidel, & Dietz, 1997). The Centers for Disease Control and Prevention is projecting that the youngest American generation will be the first to have a shorter lifespan than their parents (Centers for Disease Control and Prevention, 2012). Improving the health of our youth will require a transformation of our food systems and a change in eating habits for our youth (Fungwe, Guenther, Juan, Hiza, & Lino, 2009). The question is how can we affect healthy eating changes with and for our youth?

Increasingly, educators, policy-makers, community leaders, and service providers are finding that when youth are active participants in influential decision-making settings, they can become significant resources for themselves and others (Checkoway & Gutiérrez, 2006; Gray & Hayes, 2008). Further, it is well recognized that when young people are actively involved, they gain more from an experience, and this is a core premise of youth development and health programming (Pittman & Zeldin, 1995). As young people develop, they have the potential and the right to play meaningful roles as full-fledged stakeholders in their communities (Hughes & Curnan, 2000). Youth programs, both in and out of school, play a critical role by providing safe and supportive environments that support and increase awareness of healthy eating and physical activity behaviors (Centers for Disease Control and Prevention, 2012). This paper describes one such youth development program, the Food Empowerment Education and Sustainability Team (FEEST), as an integral part of the W.K. Kellogg Foundation-funded King County Food and Fitness Initiative (KCFFI) implemented in two ethnically diverse communities in King County, WA. In this paper, we describe the FEEST model, results to date, and lessons learned that may be helpful for others working to implement similar programs.

Program description

The FEEST began in 2008, and since then has been active in two neighborhoods in southwest Seattle. It is the primary youth-engagement strategy for the KCFFI, one of nine community coalitions supported by W.K. Kellogg Foundation's national Food & Fitness Initiative (Lachance, Carpenter, Emery, & Luluquisen, 2014). The Food & Fitness Initiative envisions vibrant communities that provide equitable access to affordable, healthy, locally grown food, and safe and inviting places for physical activity and play. The KCFFI mission is to foster collaborative, diverse leadership to create long-term, innovative strategies toward equitable access to resources and choices that promote health. The KCFFI collaborative worked with two neighborhoods in southwest Seattle, Delridge and White Center, to focus policy and systems changes to create a healthier food environment. Strategies included increasing healthy food sold in corner stores, marketing to increase demand for healthier food, advocating for Women, Infant, and Children policies, coordinating school health, and improving school food.

The Delridge and White Center neighborhoods where the FEEST program runs are very diverse and experience greater levels of poverty and its associated health problems, compared to King County and Seattle as a whole. Overall, King County is comprised of 1931,249 residents, 31.3% of which are people of color, the majority of which identify as Asian (Public Health–Seattle & King County, 2013). In King County, 22.2% of residents live with incomes below 200% of the federal poverty level (Public Health–Seattle & King County, 2013). Delridge is located on the southern edge of Seattle and is comprised of 30,296 residents, of which 46.5% are people of color (Public Health–Seattle & King County, 2013; US Census, 2010), the majority of which identify as Asian and African-American. In Delridge, 28% of residents live with incomes below 200% of the federal poverty level (Public Health–Seattle & King County, 2013). White Center is located immediately south of Delridge, in urban, unincorporated King County. White Center's population is 17,400, of which 53.2% are people of color (Public Health–Seattle & King County, 2013), the majority of which identify as Asian. In White Center, 48% of residents live with incomes below 200% of the federal poverty level. At the two high schools where FEEST is based, the free and reduced lunch rates are 60 and 82% (Washington State Office of the Superintendent for Public Instruction, 2011). More than 90% of the youth that come to FEEST are immigrants or youth of color.

The FEEST model

FEEST's mission is: "To gather young people together to prepare and share healthy, delicious food, learn about growing food, and provide a space for youth to become actively engaged in issues of food resources and the built environment in their lives." Four beliefs guide the approach: (1) Everyone has knowledge; (2) Creativity is essential to everything we do; (3) We learn by doing; and (4) We acknowledge our connection to greater cycles.

In 2008, the KCFFI approached Youngstown Cultural Arts Center to lead the youth engagement work of the initiative. FEEST became the youth development program, beginning with weekly dinners where youth cooked and ate local, fresh food while engaging in facilitated discussions around the interaction between communities and local food systems. Since those initial dinners, FEEST programming expanded to include internships and other activities (e.g. bike club, youth summit, etc.), and now occurs on site at two local high schools. The youth that participate in FEEST range in age from 12 to 24.

FEEST uses a power-sharing model in which all participants have an important voice, and youth and adults work side by side to achieve goals. This youth-driven program runs contrary to more traditional authoritarian hierarchy that is still the norm for most youth programming. FEEST's "pass the power share the power" culture builds an environment that ensures participants, both youth and adults, are aware of their privilege and power and are consciously working together to create equity while also striving to understand each other. FEEST practices are adapted in part from Kolb's Experiential Learning Cycle (Kolb, 1984), which frames experiential learning holistically and inclusive of the following: gaining concrete experience, using reflective observation, and active experimentation based on theories or ideas for action. By empowering youth to actively participate in the development and operation of the very programs targeted to support them, these programs can have a more meaningful and lasting impact on the youth involved. The core components of FEEST are weekly dinners, community potlucks, and internships. Each is expanded upon in the following sections.

Weekly dinners

The core community building and power-sharing activity of FEEST is the weekly dinner. Once a week youth leaders descend upon a high school kitchen to make a FEEST. Youth interns promote FEEST to their classmates, friends, and community; teachers and the local YMCA promote FEEST to youth they work with. All are welcome, regardless of the number. The gathering element of a FEEST, a shared meal, is made possible by donated produce from local farmers markets, food banks, and local community gardens, as well as a small budget of $50 a week to feed approximately 40 kids. At a FEEST, youth participate in (and lead) all aspects of the community meal. Those present assess the produce available and decide upon a menu, creating without recipes. Up to 15 youth can participate in cooking the meal, limited by the size of the kitchen. Those who cannot participate in the cooking, participate in creative activities focused on their own health, healthy eating, and their thoughts about health in their community.

Once the meal is prepared, the whole group eats and then cleans up together. Weekly dinners offer youth a chance to come together in a positive and accepting community to learn skills through cooking and leading. FEEST weekly dinners occur during the active school-year months and average between 15 and 25 youth participants.

Monthly community potlucks

Once a month, the standard FEEST weekly meal is expanded to bring together community members of all ages for a meal – still planned, led, and executed by youth leaders. Community potlucks offer the opportunity for youth to hone leadership and kitchen skills, and to advocate, educate, and connect with adult community members around internship projects. Kitchen interns lead 15–20 participants (adults and youth) cooking in the kitchen. Community potlucks have been used to make community decisions, view youth documentaries, engage in discussions about pressing community issues, and to meet with community leaders such as district nutrition service directors. During meals, FEEST uses community agreements or youth-created guidelines for behavior that serve to create and inclusive environment where all are welcome. These community agreements guide interactions, and all ideas and contributions are valued. During meals, youth are invited to share their ideas and opinions about the experience and what they learned. Monthly community potluck participants are invited to stay connected with FEEST through volunteering, contributing resources of many kinds, or contributing ideas for program direction. The FEEST blog documents many of these takeaways in real time as youth are invited to post about their experiences.

Internships

FEEST youth interns work on self-selected food systems projects that are shared with, and may impact, a larger group of people in the community. The internships build skills, knowledge, and leadership through visioning and experiential learning. They provide opportunities for youth to explore food systems in their communities through various lenses, including gardening, cooking, journalism, advocacy, and community engagement. Youth interns work 7–10 h a week, which does not include advocacy work and trainings. Paying stipends to youth interns acknowledges the value of their work and the internship structure helps youth to form job skills, build a college resume, and develop readiness for the working world. Interns conduct a mandatory needs assessment in order to cultivate a deeper understanding of the social, political, and environmental context of the project in their community. Ultimately, all interns learn to navigate existing systems of power and how to advocate within those systems for the desired change they seek.

FEEST, like all experiential learning programs, incorporates the core elements of do, reflect, and apply. Interns document their activities by creating a digital story, reflecting on and sharing what they did and learned during their project, with the hope they will be able to apply the broader lessons and life skills to new situations. Digital stories are typically conveyed through images, music, narration, text, and video clips, and can be powerful tools for change (Benson, Freidus, Rahimian, Sadow-Hasenberg, & Schromen-Wawrin, 2013; Gazarian, 2010). Digital stories can be used to extend the life and impact of the community projects as students use them for ongoing advocacy and community education.

Internships engage and empower youth, and communities benefit from their contributions. In order for youth to learn by doing, adults have to step away and let them "do." This has been shown to work in FEEST.

Table 1 illustrates the internships offered by FEEST, which include:

- *Project-based internships*: offered to eight youth via an application process. FEEST youth interns work in pairs in the garden, kitchen, journalism, and event planning. Interns develop and decide on the content focus on the experiential internships.
- *Build Our Own Movement (BOOM) internships*: focused on policy and civic engagement projects. Each year, four interns are responsible for planning and executing an annual youth summit attended by 100–200 youth from the community. At this summit, all interns present their projects in a digital story format.
- *Senior internships*: available to youth who have been through the FEEST internship program. This type of internship was developed by FEEST interns. Senior interns provide mentoring to other interns, write grants, and engage in public speaking based on their interests. Senior interns were invited to attend KCFFI leadership meetings and sit in on Strategic Action Teams on a volunteer basis. The senior interns provide continuity for FEEST, given their longer history with the program.

An example of how impactful learning by doing can be comes from a BOOM intern:

> Now I talk to more people and feel better about voicing my opinions. Speaking in front of people takes a lot of guts. I don't regret it. Cause I needed to do that in some part of my life. Starting now and getting used to it. It's a good skill to have. Because as [an] adult you have to talk to a lot of people in order to work with them and get your point across. If you don't do that you'll get trampled on cause people won't know how you feel. That's why advocacy is important.

Table 1. FEEST youth internship structure*.

Eight project-based interns	Four BOOM youth summit interns	Two high school senior interns
Two journalism – Write bi-monthly articles; document FEEST potluck	Civic & policy engagement focus	Mentor FEEST interns**
Two kitchen – Cook; manage budget; build relationships with community food sources	Responsible for annual summit	Write grants**
Two garden – Manage garden; conduct peer education; build garden care structure	Conduct community assessment; create & execute plan from assessment info; execute photovoice project	Public speaking**
Two event planning – Plan potluck FEEST; create & execute marketing plan; outreach (Facebook, blog, etc.) All eight engage in a civic and policy engagement focused project	All four engage in a civic and policy engagement focused project	KCFFI leadership role**

*Areas of focus for this work include: improving school food & increasing access to healthy retail, healthy foods.

**After youth have completed a FEEST internship, and are seniors, they may take this opportunity to develop an internship based solely on their passions.

As a youth-led program, the format of FEEST internships continues to evolve in response to youth feedback. For example, the journalism-focused internship was eliminated and a social media/journalism component was integrated into all internship projects.

Examples of FEEST youth projects:

- Development of new school lunch item using the new USDA guidelines: pesto pasta with turkey and spicy broccoli. The item was fed to 100 students and 100% of students surveyed liked the meal. The FEEST intern is submitting the recipe to the Highline school district to be considered for the menu.
- An intern-led school campaign to have students make one healthier choice. Six hundred students signed up for activities such as attending 3 FEEST dinners, participating in bike to school month, and trying three new school lunch items and received a "Healthier World, I Choose You" button. This campaign was coordinated with Key Club who collected the students' emails and followed up with them.
- Leading a youth summit to promote advocacy for healthier food. Two BOOM interns gathered 20 youth for eight weeks to plan a five-hour summit day and a two-hour after-party. This included an opening, a youth panel, and three workshop choices, including (1) Teen dating violence, (2) Access to healthy food, and (3) Community violence & story groups. This year's topic was "Our Stories Build the Future." The focus was advocacy. Eighty-five middle and high school youth attended the summit held at High Point Community Center. Two Washington state representatives attended. They were deeply touched by the stories students told on the topics, and asked a FEEST intern if she was interested in speaking in Olympia during session about gang violence in the community. In the afternoon session, members of the Washington Office of the Superintendent of Instruction, the King County Executive's Office, and the mayor's policy advisor attended to listens to students' stories about the three topic areas.
- Working on a school salad bar initiative. FEEST interns have conducted school assessments at two high schools, researched behavior economics studies, are creating a list of recommendations for the districts, and are creating a toolkit to engage students to choose the salad bar using the information from their findings.
- Building and interacting with a school garden. Three FEEST interns mobilized and coordinated support from administrators, teachers, and the principal to build a school garden. They procured the soil and supplies via donations from local organizations, and the interns led the building effort. Interns led weekly garden workshops. During the second year, the garden was in existence; FEEST interns partnered with a math teacher and programming was devised wherein students in selected math classes competed to design and create garden boxes for the garden. Thirty students were engaged in this process. The winning box was built to expand the garden. Up to eight students attend the weekly garden workshops. Local teachers take care of garden maintenance in the summer months.

FEEST partners

FEEST relies on community partners that provide support for the program in a variety of ways. Ongoing FEEST partners are supportive, have consistent participation, and participate in the decision-making processes. Multiple school partners, including school administrators, teachers, and district administrative offices, provide kitchens, meeting spaces, and a supportive home base for the program while also acting as mentors and a receptive audience for youth advocacy. State-level school partners provide school system and school food system expertise and mentorship, and are trusted advisors. Non-profit and county partners provide in-kind support such as space and facilities, as well as avenues for reaching out to youth and a platform for youth voices.

FEEST also maintains strong ties with a broad range of strategic partners that are called on periodically when specific support, resources, or advice are needed. The majority of these partners are non-profits based in FEEST's focus neighborhoods, or that are involved in food systems or healthy eating/active living work. They span a broad range of groups, from a farmers market to a legislative youth committee to a bicycle club. They are typically instrumental in supporting internship programming needs.

FEEST's most productive partnerships have been with agencies and institutions who view their work with FEEST as a learning exchange, and who demonstrate an understanding and value for place-based community-based knowledge and expertise.

FEEST results: youth and community impact

FEEST results include impacts for the participating youth, the impact they are having in their communities, and a wider influence that has spread to other cities.

Evaluation methods

Annual pre-post surveys and narrative stories are used to document the impact of FEEST on participating youth and their communities. Closed-ended questions ask about levels of self-esteem and abilities, awareness around food, connection to the community, and impact on youth perception of their own voice, influence, engagement, and participation. Open-ended questions ask youth to describe how FEEST has impacted them and their community, in their own words.

Narratives are collected at many points during a FEEST year, including stories and quotes gathered during monthly update calls, from annual interviews with the FEEST program manager, through review of the online FEEST blog, and via review of youth's digital stories and video of advocacy actions. Community-level changes were documented during the review of materials previously mentioned as well as the records and reporting of advocacy projects by program staff.

Youth impact

This article focuses on one cohort of FEEST youth in order to provide specific and grounded examples and quotes. For the 2011–2012 FEEST cycle, 11 youth completed the FEEST pre-participation survey, and seven completed it after participation. While small numbers of respondents do not allow for statistical significance or generalization, these results were consistent with results from previous years and were used to inform program changes and improvements. Based on the small sample size, we did not complete a statistical analysis of the data, but our conclusions from looking at the data are:

- *Pattern of overall improvement*: Improvements were made in every question between baseline and follow-up.

- *Greatest improvements in beliefs around bringing about community change*: The increases were greatest in areas related to self-efficacy in improving their community. For example, the percent who strongly agreed they had "influence over what their community was like" increased from 27 to 71%, and the percent who strongly agreed they were a person who made their community better increased from 9 to 71%. This increased awareness of larger issues around food and the need to bring about change, and an empowerment to participate in making that change happen, was reflected in one students testimony at a Legislative Youth Action Committee:

> The fast food industry is targeting students. One in three children are obese, and one in five [adults] are obese and fast food is only adding to that. We have all of these, right by our school. The lack of money students have, you can go to McDonalds or stay at school and have the less tasty food for free, it's hard for students to make a choice. For part of the solutions we were thinking about incentivizing any kind of food that provides healthy food and a cool hangout or something (so that we can have healthy food). (When testifying in front of the Legislative Youth Action Committee)

- *Youth were empowered through FEEST*: The program is achieving its goal of empowering youth through a power-sharing model. At the end of their internship year, almost all respondents strongly agreed with the statements about joint decision-making, being treated as equals, and being listened to by adult FEEST leaders. One participant noted:

> … it taught me how to cooperate with people and showed me some skills I'll need in the future. It was really hard making our own decisions… Personally, I tend to let other people take over and watch from the background, and I don't like make to decisions and it's difficult to get out of my comfort zone and speak up. It's easier to let stronger voices decide. Stepping up was a huge choice and gave me more confidence that people will listen to my opinion.

- *Changed relationship to food*: In open-ended survey responses, youth participants described cooking more with their families, being excited about experimenting with food, and looking more closely at what they were eating. As one participant reported:

> Being a garden intern for the past year has opened my eyes to all types of food in the world and it's an experience like never before. FEEST has been a big part of my life, and without it I wouldn't be who I am today, and healthy food would be bad food. But because of my FEEST internship – it opened my eyes and made me realize that vegetables taste good, are good for your body, and it's always better when you grow it!

Another participant shared:

> Growing up I loved McDonalds; I tried to eat it every day… When I got to high school I started a garden with 2 other FEEST members… I also learned about healthy and unhealthy food and I started paying attention to what I was eating and how it affected my body… I learned that healthy food can taste good, and in the long run our body will thank us, I also taught my family what I learned too… Now I try not to eat McDonalds or other fast foods.

For many participants, FEEST has been truly life changing. Of the 11 youth that participated in 2011–2012, one youth intern lost 20 pounds during the year as a result of her

FEEST participation, and she has been sharing the lessons learned with her family. A former intern went on to start a non-profit youth group at age 16. The non-profit youth group is called Start With a Garden (SWAG) and its mission is to build gardens in the community spaces in White Center and Burien, WA (swagproject.org). Two other interns have enrolled in culinary school, one of them saying "FEEST helped me decide what I wanted to do with my life."

Community influence

The impact of FEEST in the community is illustrated best by the advocacy/policy work led by youth, specific projects conducted by the interns working with schools and other community-based organizations and institutions, and the dissemination of the these efforts. Examples include:

- Two interns are members of the Seattle Mayor's Youth Commission.
- FEEST participants traveled to the state capitol to testify to Legislative Youth Action Committee, and again to meet with four state representatives and the Washington State nutrition director.
- Interns conducted two 60-min workshops around healthy eating and food systems reaching 80+ students.
- Interns were keynote speakers discussing food systems and access to healthy food, for an audience of 1200 students at Chief Sealth International High School World Water Week.
- One intern presented to almost 500 attendees during a plenary session at a W.K. Kellogg sponsored Food & Community Conference.
- One intern's digital story received regional and national recognition. The story, "Better Food for Schools," was chosen as a *Project of the Day* on the national web site www.dosomething.org, was selected as one of three winners in the "Youth Filmmaker" category for *The Next Fifty's A Story Runs Through It* neighborhood film project, and was screened at a local Seattle theater.
- Local trainings and dissemination: In 2012, FEEST conducted a local training (that had a wait list) attended by organizational leaders from youth-serving non-profits in King County, including SNAP, Age-Up, Youthcare, Seattle Tilth, Ground Up, and Solid Ground. In addition, FEEST has received dozens of request for information, from as far away as Russia. This demand led to the eventual creation of the FEEST manual which is referenced later in this article.

FEEST replication manual and training

Based on its success, the W.K. Kellogg Foundation funded FEEST to create a replication manual which was published in 2012. A team of youth and adults worked together to describe the basic concepts of how to "do" FEEST, which are the backbone for the manual. It also includes concrete tools like activities guides, intern contracts, interview tools, and pre-post survey examples. Since its publication, demand has outstripped available copies. The *FEEST Replication Manual* was disseminated to the other eight Food & Community sites. In 2012–2013, FEEST youth interns and adult staff traveled in person to six Food & Community sites across the country to share the FEEST model and conduct a training (Detroit, New York, Boston, New Orleans, Oakland, and West Union,

IA). Programs in these cities are modifying the model to fit the needs of their individual communities. This national replication manual training and dissemination has reached organizations spanning seven states and that collectively serve over 800 youth. The FEEST model is powerful and is making waves nationally.

At home in Seattle, FEEST had conducted two trainings. Highpoint Community Center, adjacent to White Center, has replicated a FEEST-like program, calling it YUM. A local gardening program now uses the FEEST model to get kids interested in gardening.

Key success factors and lessons learned

There are a number of lessons that have been learned over the course of implementing FEEST and through three years of evaluation activity that may be useful for others considering similar programs.

- *Mentors that can share power and facilitate youth's goals are critical*: This work takes an adult leader who can: step out of traditional hierarchical adult–youth relationships to "pass the power and share the power", making the space necessary for youth to lead and become change agents; provide youth with the resources they need; and participate in an iterative process. FEEST staff embody these qualities and have played a critical role in FEEST's success. The cost of not doing this is losing youth trust, losing youth interest, and losing relationship equity.
- *Involve youth in everything, and be flexible*: For a program like FEEST to work, it must be genuinely youth driven. Programming must be flexible enough to follow youth-initiated direction and changes for program improvements. There must be a willingness to change internship structure, activities, and community agreements based on feedback from interns. The FEEST director has structured conversations with interns at multiple points throughout the year. In order for youth to have a significant voice, organizations will have to change their culture to authentically engage with youth.
- *Create clear expectations*: Everyone who is part of FEEST has clear roles and expectations. When youth attend a FEEST, ground rules are set for interactions. Interns sign a contract which includes an outline of their role and responsibilities in FEEST decision-making and the power-sharing structures for youth participation. Further, at FEEST, youth can make mistakes, learn from them, and try again. For example, when youth don't follow through on their FEEST internship contract, they determine the consequences. This teaches them to communicate, face their mistakes, and grow from them.
- *Build skills through projects*: FEEST participants learn about and build their individual capacity through experiential learning that is youth-led. This approach provides benefits for FEEST youth, and their communities, has been found to be a valid strategy in other youth-programming contexts (Checkoway & Richards-Schuster, 2004).
- *Engage youth early and authentically*: Youth do not want to be engaged in policy or decision-making at the "red light" stage, where it feels like tokenism rather than engagement. Youth should be engaged at the "yellow," or planning, stage. Youth are action-oriented; they do not want to sit in discussions. To authentically engage youth, invest in preparation and planning, and change the culture of how you meet or get input. All advocacy must be voluntary and derived from youth interest. Otherwise, youth feel used.

- *Meals provide the convening platform*: Food-centric movement building is extremely powerful and can be used to support other social movement work beyond food justice (e.g. race, sexual health, anti-violence, multigenerational learning, etc.). FEEST dinners have built community across the bounds of class, race, gender, and religion. Food crosses all social strata and links us all, no matter where we have come from.
- *Stipend-supported experiential internships are valuable*: Paying stipends to youth interns acknowledges the value of their work and helps them to form job skills and readiness for the working world. It also allows students who are responsible for supplementing family income to participate. Instead of working an offsite job, FEEST youth interns are learning skills, making a positive impact, and investing in their community. Paying youth interns is a powerful method for financially and socially reinvesting in a community.

The FEEST program provides another concrete example of how youth can serve as advocates and community builders, and at the same time build their own capacity and awareness, following in the tradition of other youth development programs described by Checkoway and colleagues (Checkoway & Gutierrez, 2006; Checkoway & Richards-Schuster, 2004; Finn & Checkoway, 1998). Out-of-school or after-school youth programs, like FEEST, are forums for innovation in learning and provide opportunities to effectively engage youth. The methods and outcomes from innovative programs (Innovation by Design and the Center for Teen Empowerment, 2011), like FEEST, need to be shared with schools and in the literature, so those who seek to reform their practices can access proven, effective, and innovative ideas. The FEEST model has already been shared quite broadly, and the FEEST replication manual will serve and support future propagation of other similar groups. FEEST itself has continued since the end of the KCFFI collaborative – supported directly by the W.K. Kellogg Foundation. The long-term goal of FEEST is to bring effective flat-model youth engagement and youth-driven advocacy to as many communities as possible. The lessons learned in FEEST can add to the growing body of literature around how to successfully implement youth-driven community building programs.

To learn more or reach FEEST visit: http://feestseattle.wordpress.com/

References

Benson, S., Freidus, N., Rahimian, A., Sadow-Hasenberg, N., & Schromen-Wawrin, S. (2013). Mapping our voices for equality (MOVE): Stories for healthy change. *Northwest Public Health, 30*, 22–23.

Centers for Disease Control and Prevention. (2012). *Childhood obesity facts*. Atlanta, GA. Retrieved from http://www.cdc.gov/healthyyouth/obesity/facts.htm

Checkoway, B. N., & Gutierrez, L. M. (2006). Youth participation and community change. *Journal of Community Practice, 14*(1–2), 1–9. doi:10.1300/J125v14n01_01

Checkoway, B. N., & Richards-Schuster, K. (2004). Youth participation in evaluation and research as a way of lifting new voices. *Children, Youth and Environments, 14*, 84–98.

Dietary Guidelines Advisory Committee. (2010). *Report of the dietary guidelines advisory committee on the dietary guidelines for Americans, 2010*. Washington, DC: U.S. Department of Agriculture. Retrieved from http://www.cnpp.usda.gov/dgas2010-dgacreport.htm

Finn, J. L., & Checkoway, B. N. (1998). Young people as competent community builders: A challenge to social work. *Social Work, 43*, 335–345. doi:10.1093/sw/43.4.335

Freedman, D. S., Khan, L. K., Dietz, W. H., Srinivasan, S. A., & Berenson, G. S. (2001). Relationship of childhood obesity to coronary heart disease risk factors in adulthood: The Bogalusa heart study. *Pediatrics, 108*, 712–718. doi:10.1542/peds.108.3.712

Freedman, D. S., Kettel, L., Serdula, M. K., Dietz, W. H., Srinivasan, S. R., & Berenson, G. S. (2005). The relation of childhood BMI to adult adiposity: The Bogalusa heart study. *Pediatrics, 115*, 22–27. doi:10.1542/peds.2004-0220

Freedman, D., Wang, J., Thornton, J. C., Mei, Z., Sopher, A. B., Pierson, R. N., & Horlick, Jr. M. (2009). Classification of body fatness by body mass index-for-age categories among children. *Archives of Pediatric and Adolescent Medicine, 163*, 801–811. doi:10.1001/archpediatrics.2009.104

Fungwe, T., Guenther, P. M., Juan, W., Hiza, H., & Lino, M. (2009). The quality of children's diets in 2003–04 as measured by the healthy eating index-2005. *USDA Nutrition Insight, 43*. Retrieved from http://www.cnpp.usda.gov/Publications/NutritionInsights/Insight43.pdf

Gazarian, P. K. (2010). Digital stories: Incorporating narrative pedagogy. *Journal of Nursing Education, 49*, 287–290. doi:10.3928/01484834-20100115-07

Gray, A., & Hayes, C. D. (2008). *Understanding the state of knowledge of youth engagement financing and sustainability*. Washington, DC: The Finance Project. Retrieved from http://www.financeproject.org/publications/youthengagementreport.pdf

Guo, S. S., & Chumlea, W. C. (1999). Tracking of body mass index in children in relation to overweight in adulthood. *American Journal of Clinical Nutrition, 70*, S145–148. Retrieved from http://ajcn.nutrition.org/content/70/1/145s.full

Hughes, D. M., & Curnan, S. P. (2000). Community youth development: A framework for action. *Journal of the National Network for Youth and Brandeis University's Heller School for Social Policy and Management, 1*, 6–13.

Innovation by Design and the Center for Teen Empowerment. (2011). *After-school programs in Boston: What young people think and want*. Commissioned by the Barr Foundation. Retrieved from http://www.teenempowerment.org/pdfs/After-Schoolstudy.pdf

Kolb, D. A. (1984). *Experiential learning*. Englewood Cliffs, NJ: Prentice Hall.

Lachance, L., Carpenter, L., Emery, M., & Luluquisen, M. (2014). An introduction to the Food & Fitness community partnerships and this special issue. *Community Development, 45*: 3, 215–219.

Pittman, K. J., & Zeldin, S. (1995). *Premises, principles, and practices: Defining the why, what, and how of promoting youth development through organizational practice*. Washington, DC: Center for Youth Development and Policy Research, Academy for Educational Development.

Public Health–Seattle & King County. (2013). *City Health Profiles*. Retrieved from http://www.kingcounty.gov/healthservices/health/data/CityProfiles.aspx

U.S. Census. (2010). *State and country QuickFacts*. Washington, DC: United States Bureau of the Census. Retrieved from http://quickfacts.census.gov/qfd/

Washington State Office of the Superintendent for Public Instruction. (2011). *Washington State School Report Card, Chief Sealth International High School 2011–12*. Retrieved from http://reportcard.ospi.k12.wa.us/summary.aspx?schoolId=1099&OrgType=4&reportLevel=School&year=2011-12

Whitaker, R. C., Wright, J. A., Pepe, M. S., Seidel, K. D., & Dietz, W. H. (1997). Predicting obesity in young adulthood from childhood and parental obesity. *New England Journal of Medicine, 337*, 869–873. doi:10.1056/NEJM199709253371301

Community engagement for policy and systems change

Mia Luluquisen and Lauren Pettis

Alameda County Public Health Department, Office of the Director, Oakland, USA

The Health for Oakland's People and Environment Collaborative prioritized building Oakland (California, USA) community residents' capacity to engage in systems and policy changes toward improving food access and neighborhood conditions for physical activity. This article describes the process for community engagement, summarizes results, and analyzes lessons learned from the perspective of existing literature on community building, youth engagement, and empowerment for social change. Several dimensions necessary to build community capacity were used by the Collaborative and created the foundation for empowered residents to work with organizational partners. Evaluation findings from 2009 to 2012 provide examples of strategies that developed leadership skills and brought community residents, including youth, into leadership and decision-making positions. The Collaborative's structure incorporated opportunities for community to lead new and existing food justice programs and advocacy activities. Several lessons from the Collaborative's efforts can inform community capacity practice, such as (1) developing resources and support to build capacity for community residents to meaningfully engage in policy and systems change; (2) considering elements of collaborative structure and its processes, shared power, and decision-making necessary in partnerships among diverse individuals and groups; and (3) incorporating resources and activities that sustain community residents' participation as change leaders.

Introduction

The Health for Oakland's People and Environment (HOPE) Collaborative was formed in 2007 when several Oakland, California governmental agencies and community groups – including the original conveners of the collaborative, the Alameda County Public Health Department (ACPHD), Alameda County Community Food Bank, and Urban Ecology – received invitations from the W.K. Kellogg Foundation to jointly apply for funding as part of the foundation's Food and Fitness initiative (Lachance, Carpenter, Emery, & Luluquisen, 2014). Food and Fitness community partnerships were funded to increase access to healthy, locally grown food, and opportunities for active living through policy and systems change at the community level.

The HOPE Collaborative envisions vibrant Oakland neighborhoods that provide equitable access to affordable, healthy locally grown food; safe and inviting places for physical activity and play; and sustainable, local economies – all to the benefit of the families and youth living in Oakland neighborhoods with the greatest health disparities. HOPE's mission is to create community-driven and sustainable environmental change that will significantly improve the health and wellness of Oakland's flatland residents most impacted by social inequities. Recognizing the existing system of making and implementing policies that affect food access and the physical environment, the HOPE Collaborative focused work in three areas (HOPE Collaborative, 2013):

- *Sustainable and Equitable Food Systems*: supporting policies, programs, and practices that increase equitable access to fresh, healthy, affordable food, and investing in local, sustainable, economic development.
- *Healthy and Safe Built Environments*: engaging community members in creating changes in their neighborhoods to increase active living and social cohesion.
- *Community Engagement and Leadership Development*: supporting community members and youth to develop skills and knowledge for engaging in policy-making to create change in the food system and built environment.

Several dimensions necessary to build community capacity (Goodman et al., 1998; Minkler, Wallerstein, & Wilson, 1997) were used by the HOPE Collaborative and created the foundation for empowered Oakland residents to work with organizational partners. Since the beginning, HOPE has engaged Oakland residents in a participatory process that has allowed them to assess their own community's strengths and needs, as well as design and implement processes for making their communities more accessible to healthier, locally grown food options and safer places to live and play.

Oakland's community context

In 2011, Oakland had a documented diverse population of 391,445, with no single race or ethnic group comprising a majority. The city's population was 28% African American, 34.5% White, 25.4% Hispanic or Latino, and 16.8% Asian. According to American Community Survey estimates (2011), 21.0% of Oakland residents lived at or below the federal poverty line and 12.3% were unemployed.

Oakland's cost of living, including housing costs, is higher than the rest of the country but moderate for the San Francisco Bay Area. The costs of health care, transportation, and food are higher than in the rest of the United States. As a result, Oakland has a greater burden of persons who lack health insurance and have inadequate access to health, compared to most cities in the county (City-Data.com, 2009b). Moreover, in 2010, Oakland's violent crime rate was the highest among California cities with a population of 100,000 and above (City-Data.com, 2009a).

As such, Oakland residents face barriers in accessing safe and enjoyable places for families and children to play. The City of Oakland has over 100 parks with amenities such as gardens and bathroom facilities. However, in low-income neighborhoods, residents experience poor grounds lighting, poor maintenance and cleanliness of bathrooms, repeated infestation of cockroaches and rats, limited or no signage posting community programs and hours of operation, lack of multilingual signage, lack of sporting equipment, and the disrepair of sporting areas in local parks. A shortfall in the 1989 and 1993 property tax reductions, Lighting and Landscape Assessment District, resulted in a \$7.3 million park maintenance deficit for the fiscal years 2005–2007 and contributed to Oakland parks' decaying conditions (City-Data.com, 2009b).

During 2005–2007, three studies conducted by the University of California, Berkeley, in partnership with the ACPHD, found that residents in Oakland's low-income neighborhoods were unable to access healthy foods due to the lack of proximity to vendors that stock affordable healthy foods (Unger & Wooten, 2006). As in many other cities (Larson, Story, & Nelson, 2009), several factors have produced neighborhood conditions that adversely impact food access. For example, there have been decreasing numbers of large grocery stores in low-income Oakland neighborhoods because of city and regional planning inequities such as disparate neighborhood revitalization, gentrification, and poorly planned efforts to provide incentives for new commercial enterprises (Unger & Wooten, 2006).

In the area of focus of the HOPE Collaborative – the low-income flatlands – residents have been able to purchase most of their basic food necessities only from neighborhood convenience stores and liquor stores. As of 2005, there were 350 stores licensed to sell liquor in Oakland for a population of approximately 400,000 residents, or one store for every 1150 people. In the poorest neighborhoods, such as West Oakland, there is one liquor store for every 300 residents. Of greatest concern is that these corner and liquor stores, more often than not, sell few fresh and healthy foods and stock a limited variety of food items, most of which are lacking in nutritional value and quality (Unger & Wooten, 2006).

HOPE Collaborative's strategies to engage community residents

Following an assessment of the Oakland food system by the Oakland Food Policy Council (OFPC), a recommendation was made to engage community residents in assessing the existing food system and developing a sustainable food plan for the city (Unger & Wooten, 2006). At the outset, the HOPE Collaborative made community engagement a priority strategy. Community residents were integral to leadership and decision-making in the development and design of priorities, strategies, and programs, as well as the function of the HOPE Collaborative Steering Committee. Moreover, activities to secure involvement of Oakland's residents were incorporated in several policy and program areas. HOPE recognized the necessity of capacity-building trainings and initiatives, which have sustained resident engagement throughout the planning and implementation phases of the initiative. The following section describes specific structures, strategies, and project activities employed by the HOPE Collaborative aimed at community engagement during 2009–2012.

Create mechanisms for community involvement in the planning process

Two aligned long-term goals of the HOPE Collaborative are to ensure that the City of Oakland (1) adopts a health element to address the link between built environment and health; and (2) incorporates the framework of complete streets into the City's General Plan. Complete streets are designed so that all users (e.g. motorists, bicyclists, and pedestrians) have safe use and adequate access (Smart Growth America, 2010).

One of the strategies implemented to reach these goals is the creation of mechanisms for community involvement in the City of Oakland's planning process, thereby establishing a mandated "neighborhood" planning process that allows community residents to effectively advocate for additional usable parks, playgrounds, gardens, and green spaces for physical activity and play.

The HOPE Collaborative built the capacity of residents to advocate for the health element and for complete streets, partnering with the City of Oakland staff and the ACPHD's Place Matters Initiative. Combined, these groups have been a major influence in moving this dual-action agenda forward. Activities have included conducting neighborhood planning, hosting community engagement events, conducting interviews, and hiring two community members as team leaders. HOPE conducted neighborhood mapping sessions with Oakland's Elmhurst community residents and presented these plans to the area's Neighborhood Crime Prevention Council (NCPC) and Community Development Block Grant Board for consideration and adoption by the City's Planning Commission.

HOPE has been partnering with the City of Oakland and Alameda County Public Health Department to implement a healthy neighborhood plan, specifically for the lower Elmhurst area, to be used as a tool for advocacy in Oakland's General Plan. HOPE members chose Oakland's Elmhurst area for its neighborhood planning efforts because there were planning projects already happening in the area. As a result of the HOPE efforts, there has been an increase in civic engagement in this area. For example, three neighborhood residents have agreed to be community leaders and several neighborhood residents have participated in neighborhood mapping sessions. Results from this effort include greater community resident involvement and advocacy with their NCPC and Community Development Block Grant Board.

Create mechanisms for community involvement in ongoing decision-making

The HOPE Steering Committee was formed in 2007 during the planning phase and is responsible for the decision-making and leadership of the collaborative. This diverse group of 14 stakeholders is comprised of representatives from public agencies and community-based organizations, as well as four Oakland residents. Oakland community residents have served on the Steering Committee as its co-chair and treasurer; additional residents also co-chair action teams with an agency or organizational partner. This allows community residents and organizational partners to work together in a way that ensures input from both types of partners and fosters an equal decision-making process.

The Steering Committee holds regular meetings once a month for two hours to update, process, and strategize how to best move forward in achieving its set goals and objectives. Important Collaborative decision-making does not transpire without the prior approval and blessing of the Steering Committee. Decisions by the Steering Committee are made democratically and only members that hold elected and/or voting positions are allowed to vote. Although many Collaborative members that attend Steering Committee meetings are not elected or voting members, the Steering Committee is still an open space for them to be heard, and opportunities exist for all to become a part of the Steering Committee over time. Their opinions about Collaborative functioning are invited, included, and respected.

Oakland residents are important community stakeholders and their involvement has been a key component in the way the Steering Committee functions and makes decisions. Residents are able to provide a level of insight and perspective about the ways systems and policies function on the ground in their own neighborhoods and communities. Community residents continue to remain engaged because HOPE's work is shaped by the belief that community leadership and ownership are critical to the success of policy and systems change efforts, and they have experienced their ideas being put into action.

Conduct focus groups to gain a deeper understanding of barriers to participation in ongoing programs and practices

As part of the HOPE work, the Collaborative partners with the Oakland Unified School District (OUSD) to ensure that the vast majority of low-income students eat a healthy breakfast at their schools that includes fresh fruits and vegetables. Strategies to address systems level changes to bring this about include assessing and eliminating barriers to students accessing school breakfasts and enhancing community engagement with the Oakland Fresh School Produce Markets. The Oakland Fresh markets were created to build a school-based local food system that increases access to fresh, healthy, and affordable food for Oakland residents and promotes healthy school environments for children and families living in those communities. Each of the Fresh School Produce Markets is placed in schools located in neighborhoods with overwhelming numbers of liquor and corner stores.

To collect information regarding the progress of this work, HOPE conducted four focus groups with middle school students from the following schools: Roots International, Coliseum College Prep Academy, Alliance Academy, and Elmhurst Middle School. These schools were identified because they had lower participation rates in the school breakfast program compared to other schools in the district, and they were also located in the HOPE-targeted neighborhoods. HOPE partnered with University of California, Berkeley School of Public Health students to conduct each of the focus groups. Results of this effort revealed that barriers to school breakfast program participation exist in four major categories: quality of the food, type of food served, time constraints around breakfast, and the eating environment. These barriers are being addressed by OUSD, and subsequently, a larger percentage of students are accessing the free breakfast program at various schools. Moreover, OUSD has taken over as the sole operator of the Oakland Fresh School Produce Markets, and the markets have officially been institutionalized within the district. Community engagement has resulted in several residents that have volunteered in the warehouse. With resident volunteers, OUSD gained the capacity to meet the growing demand of the OUSD produce markets. Over the past year, the number of produce markets in low-income neighborhoods in the flatlands has increased from 12 to 22.

Partner with food policy council and other critical organizations

One way to foster economic opportunities for Oakland residents is to ensure that local policies on urban agriculture facilitate access to locally grown healthy produce. In partnership with the OFPC, HOPE gathered and analyzed existing research on policies and laws related to Oakland's urban agriculture. In this partnership, OFPC acted as the food policy arm of HOPE, and HOPE functioned as the official community engagement partner of OFPC. The systems changes that HOPE and OFPC worked toward included: (1) building a local food economy through the promotion of support towards local ownership; (2) developing accessible pathways to entrepreneurship; (3) facilitating support of a regional food shed through institutional purchasing of local food; and (4) assessing the feasibility of an Oakland-based regional food hub.

With resident participation in the OFPC, a policy advocacy agenda incorporated a community perspective. HOPE and OFPC advocated for a full-city update of zoning codes because most of the then-current zoning codes and policies were grandfathered in and were out of date. For example, an Oakland food system's pioneer received a threat of up to $3000 in fines for not having an expensive Conditional Use Permit for growing food on her personal property. As a first step towards larger policy change, a policy was passed that enabled people to grow food for consumption in *all* zones in Oakland in April 2011. This was a great achievement because community residents could then grow and consume healthy fruits and vegetables in a way that was accessible and affordable to them without risk of fines. As a by-product, this effort facilitated a collaborative relationship with the City of Oakland's Planning Department.

Additionally, the partnership advocated for a change that eliminated the need for a Conditional Use Permit, which costs $2800 to grow food, instead replacing it with a streamlined amendment to Oakland's "Home Occupation Permit" that makes allowances for certain home-based businesses. The permit process for individuals who want to grow and sell plant-based crops at a pop-up stand on-site is now a one-day process that costs $40.

Community residents continue to serve on a policy advisory group and have provided the following key recommendations for the City of Oakland's Zoning Update:

- Define urban agriculture to include both plant- and animal-based food productions;
- Allow for on-site sales, locally grown produce, and value-added goods citywide;
- Ensure affordable and timely permitting for urban agriculture operations;
- Uphold the highest humane, ecological, and neighbor-friendly standards of operation; and
- Support residents to access available lands, both public and private, for food growing and selling.

Build champions for policy and systems change

The HOPE Collaborative developed and conducted a six-month Leadership Institute for community residents that built champions for policy and systems change in East and West Oakland. The two main goals of the program were to: (1) build the capacity of residents to take leadership in the HOPE Collaborative, in their communities, and in the broader policy-making arena; and (2) provide an opportunity for residents who demonstrate leadership potential and a commitment to HOPE's work to deepen their skills in policy advocacy, facilitation, communications, project management, working in collaboratives, community organizing, broadening their knowledge of food systems and the built environment, and economic and civic community ownership.

Eleven HOPE residents graduated from the Leadership Institute in March 2012, and many of the participants applied what they had learned to their work within the Collaborative, such as facilitating meetings, providing testimony at the City Council meetings, and community organizing with store owners to sell healthy foods.

As a capacity-building activity, the HOPE Leadership Institute provided an opportunity for residents to put what they were learning into practice in specific community engagement activities. For example, a resident came into the Leadership Institute and learned new skills such as how to refine her strategies when speaking to certain audiences. Her community project with the Food Transportation Resource Connection involved organizing a transportation service to ensure healthy food options are more accessible for residents in her residential complex. She also worked together with the Food Bank so that her neighbors received earth boxes to grow produce in their homes. All of these community engagement activities benefited from her improved capacity to speak with collaborative stakeholders.

Another resident had been doing work in the community for years, well before the HOPE Collaborative was first established. The Learning Institute allowed her to build on her current skills to update the Flavors of the Garden cookbook developed by People's Grocery, a community-based organization in West Oakland that focuses on economic development and food justice through urban gardens, produce sales to local community members, and the distribution of "grub boxes" of seasonal produce to low-income families. Since the Leadership Institute, this participant has given interviews, written pieces for the OFPC website, testified at transportation meetings, and had her testimony video posted on the government website.

These examples indicate that community residents – and the work of the HOPE Collaborative – benefited from a concerted leadership training program. As a member of the HOPE Executive Committee and previous Built Environment Action Team Co-Chair, a resident who has been with the HOPE Collaborative since the planning phase emphasized, the lessons were successfully aimed at developing participants' leadership and engagement for creating positive changes in the community. As a graduate of the Leadership Institute, he reports using the communication and relationship building skills and applying them to his participation in the community engagement piece of the HOPE Neighborhood Planning Initiative.

Provide a youth lens

The HOPE Collaborative Youth Action Board (YAB) is a collection of ethnically diverse youth from Oakland, California, that originated from a larger project called Youth Building Healthy Communities. YAB provides the HOPE Collaborative with a youth lens, ensuring youth always have a voice in the system and policy changes that affect their community.

YAB created a youth-driven social enterprise program for East Oakland to help community members live healthy, eat healthy, have jobs, and make healthy decisions by learning where to get nutritious food, services, and produce. Their objective was to ensure that all youth in East Oakland would be able to easily access fresh, affordable food whenever they want and lead healthier lives. For the last two years, YAB has been meeting weekly to focus on issues important to the collaborative, specifically regarding increasing opportunities and access to healthy ways of living and having healthy habits in the Oakland flatlands, by way of a coupon book and fresh food guide.

YAB developed and implemented a healthy food and coupon book in an effort to achieve five main goals: (1) raise awareness about food justice and health disparities in East Oakland among their peers; (2) provide a resource and inexpensive way for youth and community members to access healthier foods and community gardens; (3) create a reimbursement program for local stores and gardens; (4) encourage more youth engagement with local community-based organizations and events working on food justice issues; and (5) create a new youth social enterprise opportunity for 16–22-year olds through coupon book sales and engagement in and outreach regarding food issues of importance in East Oakland.

The youth group succeeded in their project, which included compiling information on healthy eating and the location of farmers markets, and the youth participants gained skills in program planning, marketing, advocacy, and policy development. The book was distributed throughout the HOPE Collaborative and its partners, and it raised awareness about healthy food options in the city.

HOPE's efforts at youth engagement with YAB provided opportunities for youth to lead and take action on their food justice priorities. The YAB coupon book project lasted for one year and paved the way for additional youth engagement opportunities within the HOPE Collaborative. For sustaining youth engagement, HOPE's commitment to fostering positive youth development in a community setting requires an ongoing and goal-oriented process. Youth must engage in meaningful activities that build their skills and in projects that they believe will make a difference in their lives (Pittman, Irby, Tolman, Yohalem, & Ferber, 2003).

Youth are often inappropriately placed in powerless positions. Since the establishment of the HOPE YAB, it has been particularly challenging to have youth members actively participate on the Steering Committee. In a focus group with members of YAB, they reported feeling that they were not listened to or respected for their opinions. They found it difficult being around many adults because their messages and work got "lost" among the adults. YAB gave them a forum in which they were listened to, and their priorities were addressed.

Working with youth requires a worldview, considerate approaches, and engaging methodologies that pay attention to their priorities and life circumstances while fostering their long-term dedication to community change. Young people have skills in community organizing, facilitating meetings, conducting outreach, and coordinating major campaigns, as described in the YAB coupon book project. As Checkoway and Gutierrez (2006) propose, youth must be seen as resources who contribute their perspectives, skills, and life experiences in the design and implementation of programs.

Insights and lessons from HOPE Collaborative's community engagement strategies

The HOPE Collaborative made a commitment to engage Oakland residents, most of whom are people of color and reside in the low-income neighborhoods of Oakland's flatlands. These residents bear the greatest burden of the health and social inequities related to food access and poor neighborhood conditions (Beyers et al., 2009). In the process of engaging Oakland residents, several challenges emerged, including both structural and relational challenges. Structural challenges to community engagement have included mechanisms, such as committees, groups, events, and activities that the HOPE Collaborative provides as opportunities or pathways to work with Oakland residents. Relational challenges refer to dynamics in collaborative organizations that address resource and power sharing in decision-making. Reflection on these challenges has raised a number of lessons learned and recommendations for sustaining community resident engagement in complex partnerships aimed at policy and systems change.

Several lessons were learned from HOPE Collaboratives' community engagement efforts, including the following: (1) include adequate financial resources in the budget to support capacity building, such as leadership trainings and compensation; (2) incorporate opportunities for shared power and decision-making among racially and economically diverse members; and (3) ensure sustainable engagement by providing opportunities for experiencing early success and deeper dedication to the work.

Include adequate financial resources in the budget to support capacity building such as leadership training and compensation

Findings from the Leadership Institute indicate that community residents and the HOPE Collaborative benefited from a concerted leadership training program. Resources for building community residents' capacity should include comprehensive, intensive leadership trainings on community organizing, policy advocacy, and specific skills to change systems and policies related to food access and built environments. Funding for similar leadership trainings need to be robust with adequate resources in the operations budget. HOPE had originally planned for a larger curriculum but had to change it due to funding circumstances. An adequate budget for trainings would ensure that all topics and skill areas are sufficiently covered for maximum impact. A goal of the trainings should be to ensure that community residents can advocate effectively for themselves.

There also needs to be a concerted effort to provide residents with financial compensation for participation, rather than insisting that they volunteer their time. As stated earlier, the residents who are most impacted by health inequities typically have little or no disposable income. They also often have the greatest interest in and commitment to ensuring policy and systems changes in their communities. With the HOPE Collaborative, funds were available for stipends to support participation, which fostered the ability of residents to participate in the Collaborative's various projects and activities. The recommended strategy, however, is that stipends need to be coupled with strategies that ensure residents' ongoing and sustained involvement.

Incorporate opportunities for shared power and decision-making among racially and economically diverse members

Community residents often experience being at the lower end of the power and privilege spectrum. Many times, decisions at the community level are made by those who occupy staff positions in agencies, community-based organizations, and policy-making institutions.

Since there are only four residents on the Steering Committee, their voices can get lost or overlooked because of the unequal presence of organizational members. Many of the organizations around the table have been there since HOPE was first established and, therefore, have always maintained the ability to vote during Steering Committee meetings. If there are multiple representatives from one organization, then their votes all count as one. The only time transitions occur on the Steering Committee is when there are co-chair elections and new people come into those positions. The persons and/or positions with decision-making power were decided when the Collaborative first came about, and since that time, there has been considerable turnover with the director's position. There have been no transparent processes for deciding who has voting power on the Steering Committee and there is no formal process for having co-chair elections. Elections have come so infrequently, it has been difficult to get new people involved with the Steering Committee. One resident in particular has had a seat on the Steering Committee since the Collaborative was first established in 2007. Residents continue to be truly committed, and while they often have difficulty influencing the direction of the Collaborative, their opinions about organizational functioning are invited and respected.

Evaluation findings from interviews with adult residents indicated a desire for more ways to be in leadership and decision-making positions in the Collaborative. They requested more opportunities to be seen as more than "community residents" and wanted places within HOPE to showcase their leadership skills. As an example, a YAB member participated in the Leadership Institute and learned how to speak to different audiences in a way that got her point across. With these skills, she reported growing more comfortable talking to "youth about different leadership roles, how to be a leader, the steps to go about it, and how to be a leader while still maintaining lives as a teenager."

Ensure sustainable engagement by providing opportunities for experiencing early success and deeper dedication to the work

Physical and social conditions in many low-income neighborhoods in Oakland are not on par with middle-class neighborhoods as a result of divestment, similar to other urban areas of the U.S. (Anthony, 2010; Fullilove, 2004). Therefore, many community residents who have been involved in the HOPE Collaborative prioritize short-term concrete improvements in order to see immediate changes take place in their neighborhoods.

This type of priority setting was evident in the YAB food coupon project. For the youth, it was important to have concrete deliverables that could be produced within a reasonably short period of time. As a result of having short-term success, the youth's dedication and ability to push through difficulties and obstacles showed concrete accomplishments. As the youth coordinator said,

> it is important to go onto what you want, staying on target with what you can accomplish. Even though the process might be difficult, stick to your guns and push through it. It's rewarding because now they can see change from their efforts.

This is crucial to developing sustainable strategies for community engagement.

In order to keep community residents engaged and at the table for the long term, there must be a system in place to address the shorter term priority issues of the residents. Funds need to be invested so that short-term projects can be realized in a collaborative neighborhood approach. For example, it was essential that Leadership Institute graduates have specific projects and tasks that met their needs and also contributed to the work of the Collaborative.

Another important element for sustainability is to support ongoing teamwork that creates meaningful products for the community. The YAB's coupon book project is an excellent example of youth working together as a team. YAB members shared that they learned how they could do anything if they work together and put in effort. They reported that just seeing some of their efforts come to life made them feel inspired to keep doing this work.

Conclusion

This article captures a three-year window in the HOPE Collaborative's efforts at community engagement. There is evidence that the HOPE Collaborative incorporated dimensions identified by Goodman et al. (1998) that build community capacity: *participation, leadership, skills*, and *resources*. Community residents participated in program planning and implementation. Others were also engaged through the Leadership Institute and as decision-making individuals in the Steering and Program Committees. Many grew leadership and advocacy skills through active involvement in policy campaigns. Although evidence of how HOPE's engagement strategies are sustained requires further evaluation, findings to date indicate that creating opportunities and capacity for authentic civic engagement is essential to the process of community change.

References

American Community Survey. (2011). *U.S. Census Bureau.* Retrieved November 7, 2013, from http://factfinder2.census.gov/faces/tableservices/jsf/pages/productview.xhtml?pid=ACS_11_1YR_CP03&prodType=table

Anthony, C. (2010). Energy policy and inner city abandonment. *Race, Poverty and the Environment, 17*, 51–53.

Beyers, M., Brown, J., Cho, S., Desautels, A., Gaska, K., Horsley, K., & Woloshin, D. (2009). *Life and death from unnatural causes: Health and social inequity in Alameda County.* Retrieved November 7, 2013, from http://www.acphd.org/media/53628/unnatcs2008.pdf

Checkoway, B. N., & Gutierrez, L. M. (Eds.). (2006). *Youth participation and community change*. Binghamton, NY: The Haworth Press.

City-Data.com. (2009a). *Crime rate in Oakland, California (CA)*. Retrieved November 7, 2013, from http://www.city-data.com/crime/crime-Oakland-California.html#ixzz2HK09T9sT

City-Data.com. (2009b). *Oakland, California (CA) poverty rate data – Information about poor and low income residents*. Retrieved November 7, 2013, from http://www.city-data.com/poverty/poverty-Oakland-California.html#ixzz2HK09T9sT

Fullilove, M. T. (2004). *Root shock: How tearing up city neighborhoods hurts America and what we can do about it*. New York, NY: A One World/Ballantine Book.

Goodman, R., Spears, M., McLeroy, K., Fawcett, S., Kegler, M., Parker, E., … Wallerstein, N. (1998). Identifying and defining the dimensions of community capacity to provide a basis for measurement. *Health Education and Behavior, 25*, 254–278.

HOPE Collaborative. (2013). Retrieved March 11, 2014, from http://www.hopecollaborative.net/about-us

Lachance, L., Carpenter, L., Emery, M., & Luluquisen, M. (2014). An introduction to the food and fitness community partnerships and this special issue. *Community Development, 45*, 215–219.

Larson, N. L., Story, M. T., & Nelson, M. C. (2009). Neighborhood environments. *American Journal of Preventive Medicine, 36*, 74–81.e10. doi:10.1016/j.amepre.2008.09.025

Minkler, M., Wallerstein, N., & Wilson, N. (1997). Improving health through community organization and community building. *Health Behavior and Health Education: Theory, Research, and Practice, 3*, 279–311.

Pittman, K. J., Irby, M., Tolman, J., Yohalem, N., & Ferber, T. (2003). *Preventing problems, promoting development, encouraging engagement: Competing priorities or inseparable goals?* Retrieved November 7, 2013, from the Forum for Youth Investment, Impact Strategies, Inc. website: http://test.forumfyi.org/files/Preventing%20Problems,%20Promoting%20Development,%20Encouraging%20Engagement.pdf

Smart Growth America. (2010). *National Complete Streets Coalition: What are complete streets?* Retrieved March 11, 2014, from http://www.smartgrowthamerica.org/complete-streets/complete-streets-fundamentals/complete-streets-faq

Unger, S., & Wooten, H. (2006). *A food systems assessment for Oakland, CA: Toward a sustainable food plan*. Retrieved March 11, 2014, from Oakland Mayor's Office of Sustainability website: http://oaklandfoodsystem.pbworks.com/f/Oakland%20FSA_6.13.pdf

"Call for Partnerships:" an innovative strategy to establish grassroots partnerships to transform the food and fitness environments

Catherine H. Sands[a,b], Sarah C. Bankert[c], Suzanne Rataj[d], Monica Maitin[e] and Jonell Sostre[e]

[a]U Mass Amherst, Stockbridge School of Agriculture, Amherst, USA; [b]Partnership in Practice, Williamsburg, USA; [c]Community Health Solutions, Northampton, USA; [d]Department of Public Health, University of Massachusetts, Amherst, USA; [e]Holyoke Community College, Holyoke, USA

Building an effective citywide movement to transform the food and fitness environments requires the people who experience the greatest burden of health inequities to be at the forefront of this transformation. The Holyoke Food and Fitness Policy Council (HFFPC) developed an innovative strategy, known as Call for Partnerships (CfP), to build collective capacity by supporting local projects and engaging community residents in the movement to transform the food and fitness environment. HFFPC offered two phases of small grants to projects which were evaluated by a youth/adult participatory evaluation team to capture the process outcomes. Results indicate that the CfP was successful in reaching out to organizations and demonstrating how discrete projects can impact system and policy changes in the Holyoke community; however, much potential remains for fulfilling a key goal of CfP, which was to engage community residents in the movement to transform the food and fitness environment.

Partnerships and coalitions across the United States interested in galvanizing community leadership and participation in activities to improve the health of the community often stumble over a common problem of how to engage and empower community residents, the people who experience the greatest burden of health inequities. Concerned about a lack of consistent representation and participation of community residents in its decision-making processes, in 2010 Holyoke Food and Fitness Policy Council (HFFPC) launched an innovative strategy, known as Call for Partnerships (CfP), combining mini-grants with both capacity and network building. The purpose of the CfP was to build collective capacity by supporting Holyoke, MA-based projects and engaging community residents in the movement to transform the food and fitness environment.

Many community-based organizations are using mini-grants or micro-grants to stimulate bottom-up community engagement in neighborhood systems change. Mini-grants can be powerful interventions that provide community residents with quick wins, support for capacity building, and make the changes they want to see in their communities tangible and visible. When used in this way, mini-grants support leadership development, instill hope, and enable residents and community groups to align long-term goals for larger-scale social change (Deacon, Foster-Fishman, Mahaffey, & Archer, 2009; Foster-Fishman et al., 2006; Kingsley, McNeely, & Gibson, 1997; Workgroup for Community Health and Development, 2013). It is critical to note, however, that use of mini-grants can create the impression that the coalition or partnership is a grant-making body positioned to fund separate projects, an activity that could diminish the collective goals of the coalition or partnership. Mini-grants must create avenues to support work that follows the shared vision of the partnership and its goals rather than individual disparate goals of single organizations. Doing the extra work to engage community residents and groups in linking their goals and visions for long-term systems change fuels effective movement building.

The CfP approach to mini-grants supports community-driven projects that have the potential to illuminate community assets and present the opportunity for residents of distressed neighborhoods to feel ownership and pride (Kingsley et al., 1997). In Holyoke, low-income residents face above average rates of childhood obesity and other diet-related illnesses, teen pregnancy, and high-school dropout. But Holyoke also has strong, vibrant communities and blossoming community-driven activities. Bringing attention to these community successes rather than community needs is a key strategy to building lasting community engagement in food and fitness systems and policy change.

While sustaining steady and robust community engagement in neighborhood systems and policy change has been challenging in Holyoke, the mini-grant model has provided the vibrant first steps to linking many city wide community engagement efforts in long-term change-making. For lasting community mobilization to occur, partnerships must facilitate trust building through inclusion of community residents in all aspects of network building, create avenues for community residents to define together the vision and direction of movement building, and address barriers due to racial oppression (Deacon et al., 2009; Foster-Fishman et al., 2006; Kegler, Painter, Twiss, Aronson, & Norton, 2009; Kingsley et al., 1997; Workgroup for Community Health and Development, 2013). Through CfP, HFFPC maintains the priorities of building a strong network of community and organizational partners *and* concrete pathways for individual residents to become and remain engaged in improving food access and safe places for recreation. This paper discusses the foundation from which CfP was conceived as a strategy for community resident engagement that utilizes mini-grant funding strategies. Results from two years of CfP funding are discussed, which describe early successes as well as several of the ongoing and more intractable challenges of sustaining resident engagement still to be addressed in subsequent phases.

Background: fostering community resiliency

Once hailed as the "Paper City" for its position as a center of the world paper industry, Holyoke's sturdy industrial economy provided jobs for several generations of immigrants. The canals and dam remain, but the current economy and labor market are very different. In recent decades, Holyoke has suffered under a thriving drug trade, lack of investment in public and private infrastructure, an overburdened educational system, and high unemployment. Holyoke is located in Hampden County, which ranked 14th out of 14 counties in Massachusetts in all four years that the County Health Rankings have been published (2010–2013). The violent crime rate is 10 times greater than the national benchmark; 25% of children live in poverty, and the unemployment rate is 9.2% (County Health Rankings, 2013). South Holyoke, an area that includes the four poorest wards in the city, is home to a quarter of all Holyoke residents. Of these 10,500 residents, 85% identify as Latino and 88% reside in rental units. The unemployment rate in South Holyoke is estimated between 26 and 40% and the median income is $14,600, compared to $32,000 in the City of Holyoke. Only 12% of South Holyoke residents have a high school diploma or equivalent degree (US Census Bureau, 2010).

While Holyoke is an urban environment, resources such as food markets are spread out, requiring a car or ample time spent on unreliable public transportation. According to a 2008 survey by HFFPC, Holyoke residents shop either at the two major supermarkets or two discount markets; the most popular of which is located in the neighboring town of Chicopee, across the Connecticut River (Holyoke Food and Fitness Policy Council, Community Survey, 2008). South Holyoke is home to over 18 bodegas/convenience stores, whose prices (based on the survey mentioned) run an average 30% higher per pound of produce than the larger grocery stores in Holyoke and Chicopee.

In 2007, Holyoke became one of nine sites around the country funded by the W. K. Kellogg Foundation's multi-year Food & Fitness program (Lachance, Carpenter, Emery, & Luluquisen, 2014). A coalition of agency, community, and youth leaders came together as the HFFPC with the mission to create and sustain a more healthy and vibrant Holyoke through the development of programs, policies, community leaders, and advocacy relating to the food and fitness environment. Three leading Holyoke organizations, the Holyoke YMCA, Nuestras Raíces (an urban agriculture and community development organization), and the Holyoke Health Center became "co-conveners" administering the grant and sharing staff. Together with the broader coalition of partners and deliberate inclusion of community residents in the process of decision-making, they created the Community Action Plan (CAP), a comprehensive and actionable plan to transform the food and fitness environments in Holyoke with an emphasis on policy and systems change. Strategy groups composed of partnering residents and organizations formed to address the target areas: food access, school wellness, active living and the built environment, community leadership, and engagement. A steering committee of four youth, four adult residents, four agency members, and the conveners was assembled. During the planning and implementation phases of the grant, the HFFPC and evaluators tracked partner involvement, including individuals, community-based nonprofit organizations, community agencies, government, schools, and youth development groups. These relationships were examined regularly by strategy groups implementing the CAP (Holyoke Food and Fitness Policy Council, Community Action Plan, 2011a).

Community engagement: methods and program design

Implementation of the CAP began in 2009. One year later, the intergenerational steering committee, staff, and other core partners agreed that in order to tackle the numerous objectives of the CAP, a comprehensive, overarching strategy to engage and mobilize community residents was needed. One community member noted:

> What needs to happen is that folks need to get involved. You need to get people involved and then be patient with them, find a gimmick to keep them involved, and find ways for them to have ownership (Holyoke Food and Fitness Policy Council, Cross Site Report, 2010).

After a series of brainstorming sessions with a diverse representation of stakeholders from HFFPC, the CfP strategy was created. HFFPC would provide seed funding, technical assistance, networking opportunities, and an invitation to participate in HFFPC's decision-making committees to individuals and groups whose mission and goals were aligned with the CAP. In return, those groups would facilitate connections between community residents and HFFPC and increase their own capacity to engage in community building work by taking advantage of technical assistance offered by HFFPC. HFFPC would increase the reach and influence of both their formal and informal networks throughout the city, effectively increasing their capacity to build grassroots momentum for system and policy change.

CfP used an empowerment approach to community engagement, best described by Wallerstein as "a social action process that promotes participation of people, organizations and communities toward the goal of increased individual and community control, political efficacy, improved quality of community life, and social justice" (Wallerstein, 1992, p. 198). CfP's ultimate function was as a community engagement and organizing tool, guided by the definition of "community" proposed by Walter as (Walter, 2005, p. 66):

> A system that is multidimensional, involving people and organizations at many levels engaged in relationships with one another ... Community building practice seeks to engage with these multiple dimensions of community, recognizing the range of perspectives and relationships that exists and integrating diverse strategies and methods of practice.

The design of CfP took into consideration this concept of community as having "multiple dimensions" and "a range of perspectives" by developing partnerships with individuals and groups working "on the ground" with residents proposing their own solutions to problems in their community. The CfP design intended to put the decision-making power back into the hands of the residents who would be the beneficiaries of the funding and to engage partners working at many levels, integrating diverse strategies and methods of practice. HFFPC also provided technical assistance to applicants to help them develop their plan, understanding that lack of grant-writing capacity should not limit potential for partnership with HFFPC. All along the way, the HFFPC staff were the glue or "network weavers" building collaboration, seeing opportunities for systems and policy changes, and facilitating relationship building and feedback loops (Scearce, 2011).

Six objectives for CfP were established: (1) to increase partnerships with individuals and groups in Holyoke working to improve the food and fitness environments; (2) to provide opportunities for community residents to build their capacity in facilitation, budgeting, evaluation, and other skills; (3) to complete projects that were identified as "low-hanging fruit" or easy wins; (4) to honor the commitment of community and youth leaders by providing stipends; (5) to integrate and align all projects with HFFPC CAP goals, including policy advocacy and evaluation; and (6) to create a concrete path for people to become engaged with HFFPC through strategy teams and leadership structures.

In Phase 1 of CfP funding, HFFPC staff and steering committee members were invited to approach other individuals or organizations aligned with the work of HFFPC whom they knew would be interested in collaborating and receiving funding for a small project. Each project was to have a staff liaison as their contact as well as to provide assistance in completing and submitting the application. No formal selection process was held because the program was not seen as competitive, and a review team (comprised of staff, convening organizations, residents, and evaluators) provided feedback and support for the proposed project concepts. In Phase 1, HFFPC hoped to create a mini-granting model that would go beyond simply dispensing funding to organizations and individuals via a competitive request for proposals process. Instead, HFFPC also invited funded partners to attend technical assistance sessions on setting goals, identifying project partners, managing conflict, and evaluation.

In Phase 2, the HFFPC decided to open up the requests to the wider community using a more structured application process. Applications were accepted through one of four staff persons, each working in one key strategy area, who pulled together ad hoc groups of community leaders to vet the proposals using a scoring tool co-developed with the staff and technical assistance providers. The vetting process identified questions or concerns about applications and staff were asked to work with the applicant to improve their plan (rather than just accepting or rejecting the application outright). During Phase 2, due to low turnout at technical assistance sessions, staff and evaluators travelled to meet community residents and nonprofit leaders at their sites to provide these resources.

Participatory evaluation design and process

As part of the HFFPC intent to foster opportunities for community residents to assume leadership roles in all aspects of change-making, two youth leaders from Nuestras Raíces were paid to join the evaluation team for the CfP. From the outset, the evaluation team has looked to design ways to involve youth in participatory action research and evaluation as a way to reframe youth as change agents, rather than disengaged or apathetic teens, and to honor their ability to "speak their truth," or realistically describe the world in *their* terms (Coombre, 2011; London, 2007; Luluquisen, & Zukoski, 2002). According to Jonathan London, "Young people's participation in research offers a potential radical shift in the power relations inherent in the production and application of knowledge" (London, 2007, p. 508). In Holyoke, youth rarely have opportunities to be heard and for their views to be considered valuable. The HFFPC and convening partners believe youth voices are essential to rebuilding a healthier Holyoke.

A youth/adult evaluation team was formed that included two Holyoke youth residents who were enrolled at the local community college (authors Jonell Sostre and Monica Maitin), one former AmeriCorps VISTA volunteer, a University of Massachusetts student, and the HFFPC adult evaluators, Sarah Bankert, Catherin Sands, and Suzanne Rataj (authors). The purpose of the evaluation was both to track the effectiveness of the CfP process and determine CfP impact and outcomes. The team utilized several methods to collect data. During Phase 1, the youth evaluators conducted in-person interviews with all but one funded partner, transcribed, and analyzed the interviews, and discussed their findings with the evaluation team. During Phase 2, the team conducted in-person interviews with the majority of funded partners and collected written surveys from several partners who were not available for in-person interviews. Questions, developed together by the youth and adult evaluators, included: What new relationships were formed or strengthened as a result of your project? What were your goals and what did you do to reach them? What did not work as well as expected? How did your project make children's lives in Holyoke better?

In addition to evaluation data collected by the youth evaluation team, the adult evaluators (authors C. Sands and S. Bankert) led HFFPC staff through a group evaluation process after the close of both Phases 1 and 2. CfP was evaluated based on increases in partnerships, mission-aligned projects, community capacity building, and community residents involved in systems and policy change, and identification of residents/groups as part of the local and national food and fitness movements.

Results: selected case studies

Over the two phases, 24 organizations and four individuals were funded for 26 projects (four projects received two grants). Presented below are case studies of four projects from both phases that best illustrate the extent to which CfP met its goals and objectives. A description of the process outcomes from the administration of the program is discussed at the end. Table 1 illustrates the full scope of CfP projects that were funded during this two-year period and shows the variety of people and organizations that HFFPC was able to partner with, as well as the outcomes of each project.

Table 1. CfP projects funded in 2011 and 2012.

Year	Program	Partnering organization	Outcome
2011	Festival de La Cosecha	Nuestras Raíces: Urban Agriculture Org.	Community Harvest Festival at Nuestras Raíces urban farm for 2000 residents
	School garden training program	School Sprouts educational gardens	Elementary School pilots a teacher training program to support teachers to develop garden-based curriculum
	Healthy eating summer program	Sisters of Providence food pantry	Healthy eating summer program for young children
	Holyoke Urban Bike Shop	Holyoke YMCA	Expansion of Urban Bike shop, hired bike coordinator
	Youth outreach and school food mobilization	Nuestras Raíces	Peer-to-Peer outreach and mobilization with youth groups to improve school food
	Building Our kids' Success BOKS	Holyoke YMCA/2 elementary schools	Before school exercise program for 60 kids
	Youth Ambassadors	New Horizons	Exercise and nutrition program for youth
	Boot camp	New Horizons	Exercise program for youth
	Community dinner/ awards ceremony	Community member/ City of Holyoke	Award ceremony to recognize existing community leaders in each ward and supporting those leaders in additional projects
2012	Beaudoin sidewalks	Department of Public Works	Sidewalk repair and parent training program for walking school bus
	Skills training, enrichment program – STEP	Holyoke Community College	Leadership, environmental awareness, and wellness summer program for middle school youth
	Community gardens	Nuestras Raíces/ University of Massachusetts	Community-based research study assessing the impact of community gardens
	Permaculture demonstration	Nuestras Raíces, HFFPC youth	three-day workshop to teach youth permaculture design
	Empowerment club	CONNECTIONS afterschool program	Afterschool program for youth promoting healthy lifestyles
	Safe kids photo voice project	Safe Kids of WMA/ Holyoke Boys Club/ Girls Inc.	Program to teach digital photography skills and pedestrian safety to youth
	School garden curriculum integration	Elementary/middle school	School garden integrated into middle school science curriculum

(*Continued*)

Table 1. (*Continued*).

Year	Program	Partnering organization	Outcome
	Nuestras Raíces Film	Nuestras Raíces/I'm Nobody Productions	Film about Holyoke residents working for systems changes
	Bilingual recreation Brochure	Natural Resources Committee	Brochure of outdoor recreation spaces and farmers markets
	Teaching kitchen	Holyoke YMCA	Assistance in creating a teaching kitchen to be used by community members
	The dingle walkway	Peck School	Renovation of walkway: linking school facilities and sidewalk
	Community Nights	S. Holyoke safe neighborhood initiative	Monthly family fun nights in Holyoke
	Leaders Dance Club	Holyoke YMCA	Safe, recreational event for teens
	Noche de San Juan	Community members	Community cultural event
	Stop the violence basketball tournament	Community members	Basketball tournament

Building Our Kids' Success (BOKS) before-school exercise program

HFFPC has been strategizing with the Holyoke Public Schools to find creative ways to increase the amount of physical activity that students receive in the school day. The Building Our Kids' Success (BOKS) before-school fitness program is an initiative of the Reebok Foundation for children in grades K-5 who are dropped off at school early in the morning when parents have to go to work. At first, the Reebok Foundation contributed materials and curriculum, and CfPs provided the funding to train staff and parents to implement BOKS as a pilot program in two schools. In the first year, over 60 students participated in BOKS three days a week at Sullivan School and Kelly School. The goals of this program are to build teamwork amongst participating students, improve the students' grades in school, and to increase the students' enjoyment of physical activity. Students learn about different forms of movement and exercise (jumping over hurdles, sports, and running games). A student remarked, "BOKS helps me run fast. BOKS makes me feel awesome."

Because BOKS relies on parent and teacher volunteers to administer it, some schools have been challenged to find enough volunteers to cover the program. A greater challenge, however, lies in the overall atmosphere in many of the schools. School administrators struggle on deflated budgets to manage state achievement requirements with limited staffing and decaying physical resources. A recent successful district parent engagement strategy is the "full service community school" model in which schools partner with community groups to integrate academics, community development, family health, literacy support, and youth development. At the writing of this article, four schools have adopted the full-service school model and have shifted school culture towards one where parents feel regularly welcomed into the school and are involved in their children's education. The BOKS program supports these efforts of increased community engagement so that parents (particularly low-income and Latino parents who have been historically disengaged and disenfranchised from the system) feel comfortable and are excited to volunteer.

The intention of CfP is not just to fund programs, but to work towards an eventual goal of more community engagement in policy and systems changes throughout the city. In the case of BOKS, an opportunity to partner with two "early adopter" schools arose. HFFPC felt that bringing seed funding to the partnership would yield potentially long-term fruit, and it has. With the success of BOKS at Kelly and Sullivan Schools, two more schools (E.N. White and Donahue) decided to start a version of BOKS in Fall 2012 with their own funding; three associated programs have also started BOKS-inspired programs: The Boys and Girls Club, Head Start, and Connections After-School Programs. At E.N. White School, the principal committed to making the BOKS sessions part of the teachers' workday in order to make the program cost effective and sustainable, ensuring that the teachers, those who know the children best, are their BOKS instructors and are modeling healthy living to the children. After the pilot was launched with CfP resources, the Reebok Foundation decided to fund the program and provide materials in four schools.

The example of BOKS illustrates one of the more successful outcomes of CfP in that HFFPC was able to use a small amount of funding to build its relationship with the public school system by providing the schools with the financial means and staffing to achieve school wellness goals of increased opportunities for physical activity. Once BOKS was shown to be successful (and that students wanted it), it inspired other schools and organizations to adopt similar programs since they were able to see the success of the pilot initiatives and feel confident that students would participate. This has resulted in a change to the school system, as it has become the norm for schools in Holyoke to offer before-school exercise programs. Established programs have been able to find their own funds and means to support the program instead of relying on HFFPC grant funding.

Community awards dinner

Community leader and long-time HFFPC Steering Committee member Hazel Rosario was awarded CfP funding to organize a community awards dinner in conjunction with the Mayor's Office to recognize Holyoke residents who were having a positive impact on their community and to foster relationships between those individuals and HFFPC. The goals of the Community Awards Dinner were to bring awareness to the community about the positive work happening in Holyoke and to bring new community members into HFFPC's leadership core, both of which have been partially met. Two people from each of seven wards of Holyoke were recognized and were asked to share a $500 prize to fund a joint project working towards healthy food and improved fitness in their ward. Award winners organized activities ranging from holding outdoor community-centered cookouts to awarding gift certificates for the Holyoke farmers market.

The awards dinner received media attention with an article in the local paper and awareness of positive change spread through the community events planned in each ward. One award winner was asked to join the HFFPC Steering Committee. When asked about being more involved with HFFPC since the award ceremony, he remarked:

> All day! That's like asking me if I want to be involved with the well-being of children. Of course. Working with HFFPC seems like a stepping stone to working with kids more around health. I can be an instrument. Everyone knows me for that. So, why not use that to the positive? (Holyoke Food and Fitness Policy Council, Cross Site Report, 2011b).

His passion for park safety combined with HFFPC's connections and mission may be a stronger force in bettering city parks than either he or HFFPC could be independently. Because of HFFPC's sponsorship of the dinner, all 14 award winners are now familiar with the work of HFFPC, and see themselves as part of a network and movement. More concretely, one recipient subsequently applied for and received a 2012 CfP grant.

The Community Awards Dinner is an excellent example of how community partners can apply for CfP funds, seek out other partners to work with (in this case, the Mayor's Office), and use the money for a project that comes not top-down from an agency but from the community members themselves. However, due to shifts in HFFPC staff and community leadership, a final accounting of how the awardees spent their funds was not gathered, and therefore it was not clear whether the goal of spurring further community engagement activities in each ward was accomplished. This was one of the original intentions of CfP and it illustrates both the opportunities and challenges that may result from a truly community-driven project.

Holyoke Urban Bike Shop (HUBS)

Since 2010, Holyoke Urban Bike Shop (HUBS) has been a key avenue of HFFPC for engaging partners towards systems and policy change work regarding active living and the built environment. HUBS provides workshops to community residents and youths on bike riding, bike safety, bike maintenance, and bike repairs. All of these classes are coupled with lessons on health, wellness, and advocacy training. All participants are offered a path to earn a bike through their participation through the classes.

Prior to CfP funding, the program had two bike adjustment stands and one set of tools, allowing only two students to be working on a bike at a time while other participants observed. HFFPC provided CfP funding for HUBS to hire a Bike Shop Coordinator and to purchase two additional bike stands and sets of needed tools with the intention of increasing the "hands on" time participants get with bikes and supporting the overall advancement of HUBS programming. A HUBS coordinator was hired to assume the responsibilities of running the various bike-related programs and workshops. This put an experienced teacher and bicycle mechanic in charge of HUBS programming, and allowed the Built Environment coordinator to shift her focus to mobilizing residents and organizations to impact complete streets policy.

Through these instrumental changes, HUBS is able to offer hands-on learning to more students, with students working on four bikes at once. One of the winter bike mechanic trainees commented that "there wasn't a point when you didn't have your hands on a bike" and another youth stated that "they had me doing things hands-on even when I didn't want to" (Holyoke Food and Fitness Policy Council, Cross Site Report, 2011b). An adult volunteer noted that initially students didn't want to touch the bike grease that is critical to proper bike maintenance, but that by the end of the 16-week program, they no longer feared it and could use it with comfort. Overall the participants agreed that they enjoyed the workshop, learned a lot, and are proud of their new skills. The program now is funded entirely by the YMCA and its volunteers, and a train-the-trainer workshop provides a pathway for youth leadership development.

Since its initial funding, HUBS has supported policy changes to improve bikeability in the city. HUBS members have testified before the City Council Public Safety Sub-Committee; they are educating cyclists, young, and old, about the importance of cycling infrastructure in the city; and they are increasing the visibility of bikes and bike advocacy through rides, presentations, and forming partnerships with other individuals and groups working on similar initiatives.

This case study illustrates a valuable outcome of CfP in action. It has been able to make visible how the W. K. Kellogg Foundation funding is being used to improve the community in tangible ways, and to take advantage of "low-hanging fruit" or easy wins. Transforming policies and systems to better support healthy behaviors can often take years of laying the groundwork through relationship building, creating structures, and shifting cultures.

Nuestras Raíces gardeners

In fall of 2012, Nuestras Raíces approached Catherine Sands (author) and colleague, Krista Harper from the University of Massachusetts Amherst Center for Public Policy and Administration, to partner on a study to assess the impact of community gardens on the broader Holyoke community. Nuestras Raíces, a lead partner of the HFFPC, supports nine community gardens for over 100 families in the city. The goal of this CfP project was to empower the gardeners themselves to determine whether or how they might assess the impact of their gardens on food security in the city, and to suggest some methods to do so. Sands and Harper convened a research team led by two graduate students (one whose first language is Spanish) from Harper's Qualitative Research Methods class with four undergraduates from Sands' Community Food Systems class, with Nuestras Raíces assistant director, Diego Angarita, and garden manager, Felix Machuca. Together the team designed a set of eight open-ended questions and conducted interviews with eight gardeners (spanning several generations) in five community gardens. The students came to the project with an understanding of the complicated history of relationships between University and community partners, and a willingness to acknowledge the power differential that existed between them. They had an analysis of the impact of structural racism on food access in Holyoke, and were able to listen to the gardener's stories with humility and respect. Interviews were conducted in English and Spanish; recommendations, transcriptions, and photographs were provided to the gardeners.

The findings provided a broad qualitative picture of the values engendered by this program. The gardeners' perceptions about gardening and being involved with Nuestras Raíces follow these main themes: gardening enables them to continue their Puerto Rican cultural traditions and share them with younger generations, provides personal satisfaction, and a tangible way to build a stronger, safer community. Gardeners were confident that they fed many people – family, friends, and neighbors – from their gardens, but were not calculating pounds of produce harvested. When asked whether and how they might be interested in quantifying what they grow, they were divided. Most gardeners said that growing their own vegetables cuts down on food costs, but that they did it as a hobby. When asked what tools they might need to measure, they asked for scales and log books, and said that it would be necessary to decide garden by garden by majority agreement amongst garden participants whether or not to undertake measurement.

This project exemplifies several objectives of CfP. First, this project supported the gardeners by creating an opportunity for them to build their capacity in planning and evaluation. The gardeners provided the research team with assessments of the value of community gardens and impressions of whether measurement could work at their gardens. The researchers analyzed this data, made recommendations, and provided the gardeners and organization with suggested methods, including scales, report logs, and all weather poster board calculators. Nuestras Raíces has been able to take this information back to their internal strategic planning process. One of Nuestras Raíces' goals for this study was to develop methods to gather a more concrete indication of the impact of community gardens and the barter network on food security in the city and to determine with the gardeners how and whether this information would be relevant to their community gardens. This ties in directly with the HFFPC CAP's strategy to ensure that local and healthy food is available and affordable in all Holyoke communities and neighborhoods. (HFFPC CAP, 2011b)

Discussion and implications

Lessons learned

CfPs has seen several laudable successes while at the same time struggles to achieve its primary goal, which is to engage community residents to shift the balance of power and have more representation and voice in the civic life of the community. Described below are six lessons learned from the CfP process and implications for future design.

1. Organizations and individuals can be aligned under a common agenda of improving food access and fitness opportunities in Holyoke. The HFFPC fosters a network of partnerships over time that is comprehensive, strategic, and entrepreneurial. HFFPC resident, local nonprofit, and government partners collaborate proactively to end the damaging isolation of poverty and build community resilience (Deacon et al., 2009; Kegler et al., 2009; Kingsly et al., 1997). Data on HFFPC's partnerships have been collected annually since 2009 for the W. K. Kellogg Foundation's Food & Fitness Cross Site Evaluation (Lachance, Carpenter, Quinn, et al., 2014). Between 2010 and 2012, HFFPC staff and collaborative members reported an eightfold increase in ongoing partners, those partners who are involved regularly in the work of HFFPC, and over a fivefold increase in strategic partnerships, wherein the partners contribute to the work for very specific and strategic purposes. In addition, the number of individuals and organizations in the community viewed as potential challengers decreased by 75% (HFFPC Collaborative Partner data from WKKF Cross-site Evaluation, 2010–2012).

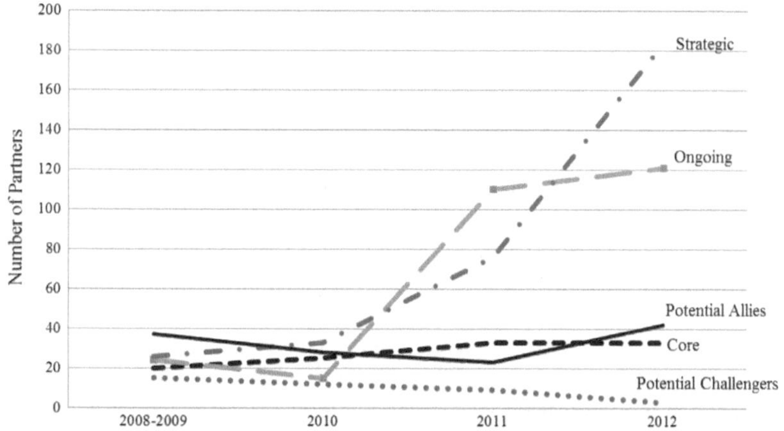

Figure 1. Change in collaborative partnerships over time.

Figure 1 demonstrates the increases in partnerships over this period. The Food & Fitness Cross Site Evaluation defines these partnership categories in the following ways:

Core partners: Central to the collaborative's functioning, involved in decision-making regarding all major actions of the collaborative.

Ongoing partners: Often present and supportive, decision-making and participation is ongoing but not as central as core partners.

Strategic partners: These partners are called upon periodically when extra help is needed for specific purposes. They are not present often but are important for particular objectives.

Potential allies: These folks are not involved but are ones that may need to be reached to advance systems change.

Potential challengers: These are the potential partners that could impede success. They have not been won over or are actually opposed to the collaborative's efforts.

The participation in the HFFPC CAP updating process that took place in Spring 2012 was additional evidence of the increase in partnerships as a result of CfP. A wide cross-section of individuals and organizations participated; 18 of whom were associated with one or more CfP projects. While the increase in partnerships cannot be attributed solely to CfP, CfP has been a significant tool that has allowed HFFPC to build stronger and more lasting partnerships, thereby increasing collective impact in systems change.

There also has been a modest increase in the participation of community and youth residents in core decision-making bodies and processes. At a Spring 2012 HFFPC meeting, one youth member spoke about how the HUBS program had taught him a skill and involved him in changing the way the city policy-makers are thinking about renovating streets to include bike lanes. He later became an HFFPC steering committee member and contributed significantly to the CAP planning process. Another community member who received a community award through the CfP project for his efforts to create safe recreation programs for children in city parks also joined the HFFPC steering committee, impacting the CAP planning process and collaborative restructuring process. The BOKS program built a new level of trust and support in the school department by partnering with HFFPC to improve the health and wellness of children. As the parents, teachers, school nurses, school food service director, and students mobilized into conversations about actionable goals, the BOKS program provided a positive visible example of children enjoying morning exercise at school.

2. The CfP projects were able to make visible to ordinary residents that change was happening in the city. Systems change is difficult to grasp because it takes so long to manifest. Systems change requires looking below the surface at the patterns and trends, underlying structures, and organization and world views about an issue (Interaction Institute for Social Change, 2012). In a city such as Holyoke, residents are anxious to see the change manifest in their neighborhood, and rightly expect grants to make a visible difference in their community. The CfP projects have provided concrete results and experiences for residents. For instance, having completed the HUBs program, young people ride away with a bike and the skill to maintain it. They become engaged in advocating for bike lanes in the city.

At the end of both Phases 1 and 2, HFFPC hosted community gatherings during which CfP recipients showcased their projects and successes through poster board displays, video, and stories told from stage. These events always included a delicious meal and provided a means for the community recipients to share their successes and brainstorm about future potential collaborations. Providing culturally relevant, tasty, healthy refreshments at community events is a key ingredient to success. Good food provides a tangible example of the kind of healthy eating for which HFFPC and partners advocate and sets a tone of sharing at events. Additionally, in a city so economically challenged, community groups and residents need resources to carry out the work they have identified to make the city more resilient. Building networks and weaving multiple strategies towards uniform goals costs money, and the progress of this strategizing is not always apparent to the public eye. These events make evident the true successes of community partner and resident programs and the power of small grants combined with community knowledge and dedication, to achieve tangible changes and outcomes.

3. The CfP program was designed as a model for community organizing, but it has yet to be utilized in a way that helps community residents to shift the balance of power and have more representation and voice in the civic life of the community. Through CfP, HFFPC has supported Holyoke residents, providing technical assistance in strategy, evaluation, and shared knowledge building. However, there remains a vast potential for engaging more community residents through this model. As CfP went from concept to implementation, it succeeded in engaging more organizational partners and supporting their immediate project needs. The goal slowly shifted away from directly engaging community residents in all levels of the process to engaging organizational partners whose projects engage residents. This trend is a common shortfall of many organizations attempting to engage in true community building work (Deacon et al., 2009; Foster-Fishman et al., 2006). The funding was not restricted only to initiatives that sought to build power with community residents; programmatic initiatives meant to provide a service to residents were also likely recipients. This may be due to a lack of capacity for understanding how to engage in community organizing where the primary goal is to *shift the balance of power* (Kingsley et al., 1997; Wallerstein, 1992). It may also be due to a lack of time on the part of staff and funded partners to work collaboratively to build community power. When people simply are trying to attend to their day-to-day details, burdened by crises and an overload of work-related responsibilities, thinking about how to create change on a systems level, particularly when it comes to building community power, can be challenging. As the CfP grows into its third round, HFFPC is in a stronger position to facilitate a more community-based participatory change approach.

However, CfP provided an opening to shifting power dynamics, an avenue for collaboration across race and class amongst Holyoke residents from different wards and HFFPC staff from convening organizations. Since the beginning of HFFPC, there has existed a fundamental tension between residents who volunteer for or are provided stipends by HFFPC and staff who are paid a salary by convening organizations for their work with HFFPC. There has been tension apparent in working relationships between staff and community leaders along lines of class, race, gender, and education or professional credentials. CfP asked both HFFPC staff and the funded partner to come up with creative ways to partner together, so that both can accomplish something bigger and better than they would have been able to do alone. HFFPC staff and community leaders are still in a process of learning how to work together towards shared goals, to trust one another, and to develop a working understanding of what it means to share power. The community awards dinner was successful because it sparked pride in residents, and bridged relationships between residents, community-based organizations, and the Mayor's office. It was successful on many levels, but the vision to engage community residents in all wards continues to remain a challenge for HFFPC and community leaders.

4. CfP, as an evolving and innovative model, was challenging to implement within a collaborative structure with staff seated at three separate organizations. The original intention of CfP was to develop a model whereby HFFPC staff, seated at three distinct organizations, could work together on one overarching strategy to engage and mobilize community residents throughout Holyoke to build a movement for change. In practice, implementing this overarching strategy has shown to be one of the most challenging aspects of the program. The three organizations often had conflicting visions of CfP and what it meant to practice "community engagement." Administrative support for the program was also a challenge, as it took a long time for grantees to be funded. While lengthy billing turnover is typical for larger institutions, this can pose a hardship for community groups and residents in low-income communities, as cash flow is simply more challenging. When this was identified as a problem to HFFPC, a new system for processing check requests was developed to rectify the problem. Lack of adequate leadership and staffing hours also was evident in that no one HFFPC staff person was able to step forward and take ownership of the program and coordinate with staff effectively to make sure that the goal of community engagement was always at the forefront.

5. Lacking a shared definition of "partnership," both HFFPC and the funded partners were often confused about expectations of the other and how to work together towards common goals. "Partnership" is a popular term used by many in the field of public health without a clear, agreed-upon definition. Without a common understanding of partnership, HFFPC struggled to implement CfP in a way that would meet its own goals, and the funded partners were confused as to what was expected from them and how they might benefit from a relationship with HFFPC. This is a common challenge for organizations convening mini-grants, as they can be mistakenly viewed as a funding entity. For coalitions or partnerships looking to establish mini-grant programs similar to HFFPC's, they must be skillful in presenting themselves as a coalition of multiple partners that have defined a collective vision that wishes to expand its network.

Initially, the staff who led the strategy groups and solicited CfP participants met to discuss this challenge. These staff members were from three different convening nonprofits. They acknowledged they had divergent definitions of level of engagement of partners, and continued to maintain that forging partnerships and mapping them for the HFFPC was necessary to building collective impact. It was also clear that improving CfP administration and designating a manager was necessary. It was determined that more could be done to engage CfP recipients in the activities of the network through invitations to participate in strategy working groups, governance, and evaluation.

6. "Building community capacity" requires a commitment to go to where people are, to meet them in their own spaces, and to do it on their timetable. During Phase 1, the technical assistance team convened two capacity building sessions on how to mediate conflict, how to conduct an efficient meeting, how to set goals, and how to conduct participatory evaluation. These meetings were sparingly attended. Moving into phase 2, the staff also approached interested organizations and residents, assisted them with putting together proposals and plans, and then later returned to interview them about outcomes and new partnerships established. This method proved to be more efficient for the partners and HFFPC, especially combined with a celebratory showcase at the end of the grant period during which outcomes could be shared and networking could happen.

Impacting systems and policy change

In the Collective Impact Model delineated by Hanleybrown, Kania, and Kramer (2012), the essential drivers of successful change-making are a combination of common agenda, shared measurement, mutually reinforcing activities, continuous communication, and backbone support. "These five conditions offer a more powerful and realistic paradigm for social progress than the prevailing model of isolated impact ... in which countless organizations each work to address social problems independently" (Hanleybrown et al., 2012, p. 1). CfP was designed to build a robust mini-grant program that weaves these elements into a framework of community engagement with real events that represent the systems and policy change happening through the combined efforts of residents, agencies, youth, and the city to achieve a healthier Holyoke. The design attempted to unite varied visions and projects throughout the city, avoiding a competitive grant model in which applicants compete for modest resources. It attempted to provide support and engender knowledge building and resiliency towards the shared goal of shifting systems through the combination of small influential actions. Community residents of all ages became involved beyond their CfP projects. For example, youth and adult residents joined the steering committee, HUBS youth became peer teaching staff, gardeners and youth participated evaluating their community gardens, and teachers and parents became BOKS trainers. The process continuously evolved and grew around the core value that inclusive shared partnership is essential. This was accomplished by reaching out, building knowledge together, achieving visible outcomes, acknowledging, and celebrating these changes with the broader community, and informing and deepening the effectiveness of HFFPC.

References

Coombre, C. M. (2011). Participatory evaluation. Building community while assessing change. In M. Minkler (Ed.), *Community organizing and community building for health* (pp. 368–385). New Brunswick, NJ: Rutgers University.

County Health Rankings and Roadmaps. (2013). *County snapshots: Hampden county*. Madison, WI: University of Wisconsin Population Health Institute. Retrieved October 17, 2012, from http://www.countyhealthrankings.org/app/massachusetts/2013/hampden/county/outcomes/overall/snapshot/by-rank

Deacon, Z., Foster-Fishman, P., Mahaffey, M., & Archer, G. (2009). Moving from preconditions for action to developing a cycle of continued social change: Tapping the potential of mini-grant programs. *Journal of Community Psychology, 37*, 148–155. doi:10.1002/jcop.20285

Foster-Fishman, P., Fitzgerald, K., Brandell, C., Nowell, B., Chavis, D., & Van Egeren, L. A. (2006). Mobilizing residents for action: The role of small wins and strategic supports. *American Journal of Community Psychology, 38*, 143–152. doi:10.1007/s10464-006-9081-0

Hanleybrown, F., Kania, J., & Kramer, M. (2012). Channeling change: Making collective impact work. *Stanford Social Innovation Review*. Retrieved from http://www.ssireview.org/blog/entry/channeling_change_making_collective_impact_work

Holyoke Food and Fitness Policy Council. (2008). *Community survey*. Holyoke, MA.

Holyoke Food and Fitness Policy Council. (2010–2012). *Collaborative partners data from cross site reports to the W. K. Kellogg Foundation*. Holyoke, MA: Partnership in Practice.

Holyoke Food and Fitness Policy Council. (2010). *Cross site report to W. K. Kellogg Foundation*. Holyoke, MA: Partnership in Practice.

Holyoke Food and Fitness Policy Council. (2011a). *Community action plan*. Holyoke, MA.

Holyoke Food and Fitness Policy Council. (2011b). *Cross site report to W. K. Kellogg Foundation*. Holyoke, MA: Partnership in Practice.

Interaction Institute for Social Change. (2012). *Facilitative leadership handbook*. Boston, MA: Interaction Associates.

Kegler, M. C., Painter, J. E., Twiss, J. M., Aronson, R., & Norton, B. L. (2009). Evaluation findings on community participation in the California Healthy Cities and Communities program. *Health Promotion International, 24*, 300–310. doi:10.1093/heapro/dap036

Kingsley, G. T., McNeely, J. B., & Gibson, J. (1997). *Community building – Coming of age*. Baltimore, MD: The Urban Institute.

Lachance, L., Carpenter, L., Emery, M., & Luluquisen, M. (2014). An introduction to the Food & Fitness community partnerships and this special issue. *Community Development, 45*: 3, 215–219.

Lachance, L., Carpenter, L., Quinn, M., Wilkin, M. K., Green, E., Tsuchiya, K., … Clark, N. M. (2014). Food & Community: The cross-site evaluation of the W. K. Kellogg Food & Fitness community partnerships. *Community Development, 45*: 3, 227–239.

London, J. K. (2007). Power and pitfalls of youth participation in community-based action research. *Children, Youth and Environments, 17*, 407–432.

Luluquisen, M., & Zukoski, A. (2002). Participatory evaluation: What is it? Why do it? What are the challenges? *Community Based Public Health Policy and Practice, 5*. Retrieved from http://depts.washington.edu/ccph/pdf_files/Evaluation.pdf

Scearce, D. (2011). *Connected citizens: The power, peril and potential of networks*. Miami, FL: John S. and James L. Knight Foundation, Monitor Institute. Retrieved from https://knight.app.box.com/shared/ng70lqn9hb

U.S. Census. (2010). *American FactFinder*. Washington, DC: United States Bureau of the Census. Retrieved October 17, 2012, from http://factfinder2.census.gov/faces/nav/jsf/pages/community_facts.xhtml

Wallerstein, N. (1992). Powerlessness, empowerment, and health: Implications for health promotion programs. *American Journal of Health Promotion, 6*, 197–205. doi:10/4278/0890-1171-6.3.197

Walter, C. L. (2005). Community building practice: A conceptual framework. In M. Minkler (Ed.), *Community organizing and community building for health* (2nd ed., pp. 66–78). Piscataway, NJ: Rutgers University.

Workgroup of Community Health and Development. (2013). Community toolbox: Establishing a micro grant program. Retrieved from http://ctb.ku.edu/en/table-of-contents/finances/invest-in-community-resources/microgrant/main

Relationship building: the art, craft, and context for mobilizing the social capital necessary for systems change

Mary E. Emery[a] and Corry Bregendahl[b]

[a]*Sociology and Rural Studies, South Dakota State University (SDSU), Scobey, Brookings, USA;*
[b]*Leopold Center for Sustainable Agriculture, Iowa State University, Ames, USA*

Much has been written about the importance of relationship building and collaboration in community and policy change work. Yet, we know little about the process of successfully building relationships in this context. The Northeast Iowa Food and Fitness Initiative (FFI) is one of nine Kellogg-funded community change initiatives targeted at increasing access to healthy food and fitness activity. Using data collected from interviews of FFI leadership team members, we deconstruct the relationship-building process to focus on the iterative nature of social capital development and the impact of this process on generating additional assets in cultural, human, and political capital to create a spiraling-up process. The resulting merging of bonding and bridging social capital into generative social capital fashions resilient ties that span boundaries and expand the radius of trust.

Introduction

Currently, over $3 billion philanthropic dollars, (Jagpal & Laskowski, 2013) as well as substantial federal dollars in the United States focus on community change initiatives with implied social justice/equity goals. Social justice philanthropy funds work for structural change that increases the opportunity of those who are the least well off politically, economically, and socially (Coke et al., 2009). Policy change is often a chief goal of social justice philanthropies to demonstrate that changes have been institutionalized to benefit the target populations and will outlive active champions. Additional philanthropic and government funding has focused on evaluating these efforts to determine what success looks like and what factors contribute to success in these ventures. This article will contribute to that discussion with the aim of expanding our understanding of the role of social capital in successful community change efforts that also result in policy change.

In 2007, the W.K. Kellogg Foundation (WKKF) invested in multi-year demonstration projects with inherent social justice goals related to addressing race and equity targeted at creating vibrant communities with equal access to affordable, healthy, locally grown food, and safe and inviting places for physical activity and play (Lachance, Carpenter, Emery, & Luluquisen, 2014). Nine communities across the country were selected to become models for change. WKKF funding supported the formation of local collaboratives to improve the health and quality of life in communities via transformation of food and fitness environments through systems and policy change (Kellogg Foundation, n.d.).

As with many community change initiatives, collaboration was both a condition for participation and an expected outcome of the WKKF's investments. Northeast Iowa, with a regional focus on the six northeast counties of Iowa, has shown success in sustaining an ongoing collaboration with few changes in key leadership, resulting in a stable project development process. Developing an understanding of how and why collaboration has worked well in the Northeast Iowa setting offers insights into the process of successful coalition building that fosters policy change, particularly policy changes at the school district/building and county/city levels in providing alternatives and/or incentives that increase access to healthy foods and fitness activities.

As the Aspen Institute found in their 10-year study of community change initiatives, "Where communities and public systems have developed effective and mature working relationships, the actions and capacities that led them there should be analyzed. This must be a priority for the next generation" (Kubisch, Auspos, Brown, & Dewar, 2010, p. 147). In this paper, we seek to contribute to this analysis and to suggest a model for designing, implementing, and evaluating a relationship-based strategy to monitor and lobby for policy change.

The importance of relationship building and collaboration in community change work

As in the case with the WKKF Food & Fitness Initiative, collaboration is a critical component to any community change work (Walzer, 2012). Glickman and Servon (1998), and Gittell, Newman, Bockmeyer, and Lindsay (1998) emphasize the participation of individual community members in a process of relationship building, community planning, decision-making, and action as key to successful social change work. In describing a "coherent approach to healthy cities," des Villes-Sante and Dooris (2009) list key relationship-related activities such as support for grassroots community-level development, the establishment and strengthening of networks, and commitment to meaningful organizational development. Community organizing and empowerment models also emphasize the development of relationships for collective action (Beck & Purcell, 2013). In their extensive review of community change initiatives, the Aspen Institute identified key lessons related to the importance of effective management of partnerships and collaborations, including the development and management of a "complex web of relationships," requiring "significant time as well as political, social, and economic capital" (Kubisch et al., 2010, p. viii).

Indeed, relationship building is so critical that philanthropies have taken note of a piece by Kania and Kramer appearing in the 2011 winter edition of the Stanford Social Innovation Review. In their widely influential piece, Kania and Kramer state that "The expectation that collaboration can occur without a supporting infrastructure is one of the most frequent reasons why it fails" (2011, p. 40). Relationship building and the maintenance of these connections require significant investments of time and therefore money. Without ongoing support, they can become brittle or break off entirely.

Relationship building, collaboration, and social capital

Multiple forms of relationships or social capital play a key role in community change work, including the strong ties that build trust and the weak ties that expand opportunities (Granovetter, 1973). Relationships create the trust that helps people work together; they provide access to information and resources, and they can link us to sources of power (Popp, MacKean, Casebeer, Milward, & Lindstrom, 2013). According to Chazdon and Lott (2010), successful leadership development incorporates social capital and relationship building in three ways: relationships that (1) bond like-minded people together and build trust, (2) bridge people with varied backgrounds and/or interests to other types of groups and organizations, and (3) link people and organizations to resources and information outside the community. Turner (1999) also emphasized the importance of linking or extralocal types of relationships or political capital, especially in regard to policy work and developing relationships outside the partnership to build political will. For some, increasing social capital through focusing on collaboration within the community also has the goal of changing the norms or culture of the community (Flora & Flora, 2012; Perkins, Hughey, & Speer, 2002; Putnam, 1995) and in expanding the radius of trust (Fukuyama, 1995).

The concept of social capital, however, is often contested, particularly in regard to its role in community change work where some view social capital as an attribute of the social system, and others view it in relation to an individual's connections. Considering the role of social capital in community change work requires us to rethink common definitions of social capital as a vehicle for exchange (Coradini, 2010, p. 576), or a resource that reinforces social difference or "alternatively, a pedagogical increment that contribute[s] to school performance, human capital and social control and integration" (Coleman, 1988; Coradini, 2010). In these definitions, social capital facilitates exchanges, either to reinforce class privilege or to provide a public good, (Coradini, 2010) much like a transfer station. Portes (2000, pp. 3–4) describes elements of Bourdieu's (1986) concept of social capital as relationships that "allow individuals to access resources." Further, he comments that the "acquisition of social capital requires deliberate investment in both economic and cultural resources." In this context, the fungibility of social capital is linked to markets and "accumulated human labor" (Coradini, 2010, p. 4). Reducing the social capital, described in the interviews and evaluations of community change work, into strictly economic or market mechanisms misses the key role social capital plays in community-based efforts that invest existing social capital assets to grow other assets. The results of our study indicate that an intentional approach to accessing and building stocks of social capital can have a transformative rather than a transactional effect in community change work.

Methods

In preparing for the research, we asked leaders of the Northeast Iowa Food and Fitness Initiative (FFI) group what focus we should take in researching the process in which they engaged and the impact of their collaboration. All agreed they wanted to dig deeper into the critical role of relationship building. Is there a coherent story to their experience in creating and maintaining relationships or just pieces that fit into another story, they asked. What is the role of relationship building in policy change work?

This research is informed by participatory action research principles (Stoecker, 1999). While FFI members were not active in collecting and analyzing the data, the focus of this research emerged from a conversation between the evaluation team and the FFI leadership about participating in this special issue. The resulting discussion focused on what reflective activity would be most beneficial to understanding successful policy change work. Thus, FFI leadership participated in the design of this research, which centers on relationships and relationship building within an initiative intended to change policies related to promoting healthy behaviors. This focus also reflects a common theme in regular conversations between project team leaders and the evaluation team. FFI leaders were most interested in what we can learn together that would allow them to act on results and to share the wisdom they are developing around successful community change work. The topics that the FFI leadership group were most interested in learning about were the factors people thought contributed to successful relationship building and collaboration, barriers to collaboration, how the team spanned boundaries (related to linking to outside organizations and groups), and the relationship of these factors to successful policy change.

Initiative members helped to construct the interview questions and approved the final list of open-ended questions submitted to the IRB at South Dakota State University. The research design was framed using Appreciative Inquiry (Cooperrider, Sorensen, Yaeger, & Whitney, 2001) with the hope that knowledge of what is working well can be carried forward to increase the success of their policy change work.

As a result, 10 interviews were conducted using a convenience sample. That is, potential interviewees were suggested by FFI leaders and key stakeholders. We interviewed the first 10 who were able to give us their time in the weeks set aside for data collection. The last several of these interviews, while providing insightful comments, did not add new ideas, leading us to believe we have reached a saturation level with the sample. Interviews were line coded to identify key themes.

Findings

Overall, the interview responses were of two types: some respondents were very introspective and reflective of the process and had many insights into the process of relationship building, while others tended to concentrate on the concrete actions required to build relationships and initiate policy change. These categories of responses reflect the participation of both abstract and concrete thinkers on the leadership team. Data from interviews are summarized below and fall into the following categories: factors that contribute to successful relationship building, strategies for building strong relationships, successful boundary spanning, barriers to successful relationship building, relationships and policy change, and advice for others.

Factors that contribute to successful relationship building

When asked how you know if a relationship is going to work out, one respondent said, "I don't know if you ever truly know. You just have to take a leap of faith sometimes." Yet, respondents identified six key factors that contributed to successful relationship building within FFI. They include trust, alignment, intentionality, diversity, readiness, and persistence.

1. Trust: Every interview mentioned trust at some point as a critical factor underlying successful relationship building.

> Trust is a huge thing. I think that we have really tried to work on creating a safe environment where you can be trusted; you can trust others and share openly without being afraid or intimidated about your thoughts.

Trust also means relying on partners with whom you work not to exploit or otherwise misappropriate shared ideas or information. Another respondent commented on the process that evolved to support the development of trust among participants, "It's not just a one-way conversation, they also share in that conversation, so I think when we see that they stepped forward with their communications and their values and their relationships, we can see that trust forming." The development of trust means that norms of reciprocity are in place and functioning.

Several respondents also talked about the importance of "positive participation on a consistent basis" as important to the trust building process.

> On an individual and an organizational basis that is very important for the individuals who are participating in such a process to be present at the meetings, to be present in all the conversations. That has done a tremendous amount for the relationship building.

Another respondent commented "I think it becomes important when they are personally asked and involved."

Trust is also important to the process of passing on the leadership roles.

> ... new [partners] will come along so we just have to trust that we have done a good enough job while laying the foundation that they will get interest[ed] in continuing [the work], and that it will evolve to meet the needs of the next year. So, when is there enough trust? I think there is enough trust when the people who were in the position initially are ready to allow it to become what it is going to become.

Thus, trust can grow and thrive when partners are committed to working toward a common agenda, as opposed to working only toward what is best for their own organization. Having a primary commitment to a common agenda does not preclude, however, a secondary commitment to organizational goals.

2. Alignment: Another factor mentioned often was alignment. Several respondents focused on the need for all participants to see how moving the work of FFI forward would also move the work of their organization forward. "There has got to be a win-win." Another respondent added the notion of working as a team, "I think partnerships come from open and honest communication, from working as a team, solving problems together, from listening." Alignment of purpose, goals, and strategies is essential as is "listening to their feedback, and then proceeding on and making them feel like what they had desired had been listened to and had been acted on."

3. Intentionality: Another common theme articulated by respondents is the need to plan how to create an environment that will encourage people to see the value of participation. "I have never been involved in anything that has had such an intentional partnership building as a fundamental piece of it." FFI was also very intentional in their outreach efforts and strategies to bring in new partners.

> Within the two years of the planning grant, [we] were able to bring together stakeholder groups and offer opportunities for them to come together to a central location, but [we] would also go directly to those people. So, a lot of time was spent just meeting in small group settings and one-on-one meetings explaining the roles of different people.

4. Diversity: several respondents spoke about the importance of having people from different backgrounds with different perspectives involved in system change work:

> When [we] went into the fitness aspects, there was a broad variety of people from all parts of the society whether they came to the meeting because they were curious, or because they were asked to come as a representative of something. We have a very wide variety from

> the civil engineers to the representatives of the hospital to the representatives of schools to the representatives of the park districts all trying to figure out how all of these different things relate to a better environment to live in.

Another commented "I see lots of different people with lots of different textures being very involved. It was very, very good … well, it was fun to be at too."

5. Readiness: A number of comments focused on readiness in certain areas, "We are noting that there's just not a readiness there. So, we're just going to back off and see in a few months or so whether there might be some readiness at that point." Assessing readiness gave them an option to determine best strategies for working with a new partner and to come back later rather than cut ties when the time was not right for a collaborative effort.

6. Persistence: A number of respondents also focused on the need for persistence. "Our motto has always been more about approaching [the work] through different avenues, so you're always trying [different strategies] for some success." Another respondent commented on viewing the work as providing "leadership with early childhood providers and educators in the region and engaging them in a regional learning community regarding what they really want to create."

Persistence also related to the amount of time and effort that building strong relationships takes at the beginning of the effort.

> … over the period of the first year, year and a half, the organizational structure [we] used and the fact [we] met as a regional group, and people came from different locations, and [we all] have different style meetings and interactive activities … led [us] to be a cohesive group.

Project leaders commented many times that a big part of their time was taken up meeting with people over and over again to help them determine if they wanted to be part of FFI. "So I think that was certainly a unique aspect of what [we] had to achieve – to get a group that wasn't used to working together to work together." Another commented:

> It requires time – where that individual is, and what is it that they are seeking from the relationship, and how can we find common ground or common understanding with the work that we're doing. That isn't always an easy thing to convey because people are being introduced to our work and thinking it's a program [as opposed to a community change initiative].

Strategies for building strong relationships

Respondents described how an intentional approach to relationship building was developed and implemented. Training in building "quality relationships" was important. On applying the training, the core team learned to work together in a new way. Through that work, they developed a way of being together.

> One of the challenges at the beginning was to figure out how to, and when to evolve. There was a lot of moving and encouragement and explanation and coaching. We decided to make a concerted effort not to intentionally alienate [anyone]. Recognizing that there is always more than one side is an important thing, and [you need to show] you [are making] a real effort to assure people that this is not meant to be opposing, but rather to bridge gaps rather than create them.

Together they developed what one respondent referred to as a brand.

> [The group] was a brand new entity, and somebody had to establish credibility before [we] could go out and ask groups outside the group to listen to [us]. [We] first had to become experts in [our] field or at least be recognized for bringing something to the table, in order to be listened to and that took some time. But in the end, I think it worked quite well for [us]. This gave us a way to reach out and be considered a resource.

Every interview included some reference to the importance of open, honest, and transparent communication within the collaborative as well as with those organizations considering joining or invited to join the collaborative.

> And once [people representing those organizations] started talking to each other, they started to recognize that even though they may not share exactly the same goal with the person sitting next to them, those goals are related if the ultimate goal was to increase opportunities for everybody to make a place that is for all of them.

The best way to do this was to frame the work as "for" the community instead of work "against" threats to the community. As one respondent commented "[By] looking at addressing urgent issues instead of getting into a problem-solving mode in our discussion, we really facilitated more of a generative discussion around the vision and the communities that we wanted to create." Another respondent commented: "Everything we say and do reflects our work, so we really need to be conscious of how we present ourselves." Positive, consistent messaging was considered essential to that end.

Successful boundary spanning

Boundary spanning is often seen as a critical element for sustainable systems-level change (Earl, Carden, & Smutylo, 2001). Community change work makes a difference in terms of who works together and how change occurs. Successfully spanning boundaries and working across isolated silos is essential for community-level change impacts. The interviews provide some insights into this aspect of relationship building for successful community and policy change.

> FFI was a team-building kind of a thing in the first place, but after [we] reached out beyond the team to try to have an impact, then I think it was about being sensitive to each group's unique place in the world. Schools are different than cities, cities are different than counties, and those groups are totally different. So, each group that FFI approached, [we] had to learn about that group and what that group's needs were in order to be sensitive to how [we] asked for their time.

And,

> We've worked very hard on [crossing] boundaries related to county lines and school districts and helping everyone see the collective regional benefit. If we've tried something in one community and take what we've learned from it into our planning, that's also [built] on a platform of trust and transparent communication.

Several interviewees commented on the range of relationships with boundary partners from those who are surface partners to those who become part of FFI's deeper core, elucidating the struggle to balance supporting the common agenda with supporting the goals of a represented organization. Regarding the latter:

> It has been difficult to have that partnership be anything more than somewhat of just a surface partnership; it doesn't go very deep. And that's what I say with a lot of our partnerships. It's more that [those partners are asking] "how is this going to benefit me? Benefit the institution that I work for?" [Those partners don't want] to get involved and go deeper.

In other words, they are not committed to a common agenda. In contrast, when the relationship develops in a generative way,

> It's really around this idea of community self-determination, and so for every new voice or every new organization, that is introduced or wants to be engaged, it's this mutual exploration around what our work is and what their interests are and, what does the fit look like within grassroots, community driven models. It's very messy and it's non-linear.

Successful boundary spanners are "able to see things from different perspectives and willing to go out of their comfort zone to learn about opportunities to achieve a larger common goal."

Barriers to successful relationship building

In responding to the question about barriers to relationship building, we heard a dominant theme. Just as respondents focused on the need for consistent participation in successful relationships, many commented on the changes in people's situations and motivations impacting existing and evolving relationships. In the following quote, the respondent reflects on his/her overall experience with relationship building and community change work outside the FFI and the importance of building capacity that extends beyond a few key people.

> We've seen time and time again that there is a key individual or a handful of key individuals who ARE the effort and when those key individuals leave, the activities die out pretty quickly.

In contrast, the FFI experience was described as:

> It's very invested within that group that it's not one individual or a handful of individuals, there's a nice cross section. If one of those people would leave, the water would fill in very quickly – that's because of that planning and that relationship building that happened initially.

Relationships and policy change

We also asked respondents to comment on how their efforts in building relationships have impacted their ability to change policy. "It's extremely important. [We] have to have the awareness of the opportunities, [we] have to be motivated; there has to be a certain level of collaboration, [and] we have to share common language." Another commented:

> I think without relationships you really can't have systems change work. You have to have a quality relationship; you have to see that shared vision. [All] parties have to be willing,

> to be compelled, to work towards that vision. They have to invest, but everyone needs to be a part of it at whatever level they can.

Still another linked the work of the first two years in planning and creating relationships to the FFI's ability to work successfully in the policy environment.

> [The planning phase] has been invaluable as we have moved forward. It was very, very methodical, and to some people, way too slow, but we always knew that you needed to go slow to go fast, and what we've seen, what happened in those first two or three years, has provided a foundation for us to build so many other things on.

A team member described how relationships can lead to policy change as:

> [Relationships are] huge. To change a policy means you have to take something that has been built into the fabric of what someone has already been doing and change it or add to it. So, if you don't understand what it is that created that fabric in the first place, then you don't understand why they have that fabric or their feelings and emotions behind it.

Another commented "Relationships are the only thing that can topple money, but it takes so many relationships to topple a relatively small amount of money. That is very difficult to do." As a former program officer in the WKKF puts it, to change policy, you need to represent the "money" or the "many" (Salvador, 2014). In this work, we have more "many" than money. Relationships marshaling social capital make the "many" goal possible.

Advice for others

When we asked for advice on relationship building, we learned about the importance of so-called "soft" skills: people skills, being able to read people, changing "mental models" and norms about the way people think, "frequent and ongoing communication," being creative and "recogniz[ing] the interconnectedness between all thing," open mindedness, "recogniz [ing] history is something to learn from," and being "open to questions and dialog as it comes up." Respondents also mentioned "honoring every participant's time" and "kids are key to involving adults." Another summed it up as:

> Entering into this "smaller" relationship and knowing that if the foundation around the relationship expands and grows and deepens, that [partners] can be exposed and take on more [relationship building responsibility] as the journey proceeds. There is such a temptation to want to tell [new partners] the whole story; but it's nearly impossible to do in the early conversation.

Throughout the interviews, respondents focused on the time and effort required to do serious relationship building work.

Discussion

The data describe a complex interaction among social, human, cultural, and political capital. The mobilization of existing assets in social capital led to increased assets in other capitals as the process of relationship building unfolds. Indeed, these data can help us unpack the spiraling-up effect (Emery, Flora, Gutierrez, & Fernandez-Baca, 2006) by demonstrating how assets in one capital (social) can be transformed into other forms of capital (human and cultural), expanding the stock of assets available to support community and policy change work. Reflecting on the data and on the results of other evaluations of successful change work (Fulbright-Anderson & Aupos, 2006), the value of bonding and bridging social capital in this work becomes clear.

Yet, the interviews speak of something beyond building trust and accessing resources and information. In examining the data, we see an iterative pattern of bonding and bridging social capital, which at the same time produces new assets in cultural (Keating & Gasteyer, 2012) and human capital and eventually political capital.

For the purposes of this discussion, we can distinguish the results of this relationship building process as *generative social capital* to differentiate this formation of social capital from the market-like exchange of resources. Generative social capital is not an exchange; it has generative properties that lead to new configurations in the intangible capitals and that initiate the spiraling-up or virtuous cycle critical to successful and sustainable community and policy change work.

The interview data provide insight into how this process works. At the initial stage, initiators of the process listened to each other, told their stories and shared ideas, thus creating a common purpose and the trust needed to work together. They created new assets in human capital in the form of place-based knowledge and new elements of cultural capital in defining new ways of thinking and doing in relation to their purpose. Together they created a different way of working together. The interviews described a process that was open to any who wanted to participate in working toward a healthier community. From these conversations, they developed a leadership team and steering committee that focused on planning. They put resources into this aspect of their work with the premise that relationship building and trust would lead to better collaborative and cooperative thinking that would result in more effective collective action. They developed their own theory of change around relationships and trust leading to collective action and successful policy change work.

The group also accessed bridging social capital by participating in Kellogg-funded training, which led to the creation of bonding social capital with "outsiders," thus expanding the radius of trust (Fukuyama, 1995) leading to additional growth in human and cultural capital. In this case, the focus on taking a systems approach to community and policy change impacted the everyday ways of thinking and doing within the group and the initial partners. As new partners were brought in, they also contributed to generating new knowledge and expanding bridging social capital, often leading to surprising results. Thus, human capital increased as contact with different organizations and people expanded the overall knowledge and understanding of the community.

Participation within FFI led to increased bonding social capital with new participants, and access to their networks expanded the stocks of bridging social capital. At the same time, participation in the expanding partnerships led both to new insights and access to additional information and resources. This iteration of expanding bonding and bridging capital among new partners led to the "new habits of thinking, acting, and collaborating [that] enable these alignments to occur more naturally" that Kubisch et al. (2010, p. 77) determined were essential in successful community change efforts.

Generative social capital, and the processes it facilitates, is not linear; it is about changing the mental models critical to real system-level change. The relationships evolved as partners found ways to support the effort at the same time they supported each other. Sometimes this process required FFI members to return again and again and show tangible results during the process of building strong relationships with new partners.

Often this work is categorized as building bridging social capital with its focus on the strength of weak ties (Granovetter, 1973). Yet, the resulting relationships are not bridging/weak ties nor bonding/strong ties in the community change work; the result is a both/and rather than an either/or. These connections are transformed into a hybrid of resilient ties that span networks and not only provide access to resources, but are also able to build trust across the networks of weak ties. Thus, the strength of weak ties is multiplied and the radius of trust can expand exponentially (Fukuyama, 1995). The function of building and maintaining relationships among community actors and between the community and external actors – especially businesses and public agencies – is one that needs to be lifted up as a key component of community change work (Kubisch et al., 2010, p. 182).

The development of generative social capital means that people learn to work across silos and in different contexts such that "relationships that motivate action and create collective accountability" (Kubisch et al., 2010) build a foundation for successful policy change work.

Toward a model of generating generative social capital by focusing on relationship building

The FFI experience provides an example of an intentional approach to relationship building as a foundation for engaging communities and organizations in successful policy change work. Drawing on the results of the interviews and the key points identified by respondents, an emerging model for relationship building that creates and mobilizes generative social capital includes an intentional design state, a focus on learning through implementation, and incorporating evaluation throughout. This model also requires a commitment of time and financial resources to the long-term goal of building relationships.

(A) Designing for change: The planning team developed a format for bringing people into the work of the initiative from the beginning as actors rather than participants, which included four key tasks:

(1) Focus on the purpose; develop the brand to help others understand what you bring to the table.
(2) Plan to move slowly to engage all members in determining direction and developing new ways of thinking and doing.
(3) Organize the work to uncover tacit knowledge about the situation and privilege the resulting local wisdom over outside and expert knowledge; use outside knowledge and coaching strategically to build new relationships and generative approaches to local issues.
(4) Hold the door open for those who have an interest in joining the effort and encourage them to plug in where and when they can.

(B) Implementing for change: As the plan unfolded, FFI was mindful of each of the following tasks:

(1) Retrace the work around direction and renew and maintain relationships regularly.
(2) Expand the work through intentional connections with organizations and agencies.
(3) Bring in new partners slowly by engaging them informally to both learn from them and to identify possible areas for alignment; revisit regularly.
(4) Integrate reflection to learn from each other and create new insights into the work of policy change formally in meetings and regularly with staff and key partners.

(C) Evaluating for change: The FFI experience also provides guidance in measuring the success of relationship-building goals and activities:

(1) Focus evaluation on relationships among people and organizations over time and on what happens as a result of those relationships.
(2) Use reflexive approaches to understand not just what is happening but why.
(3) Focus on organization, community, and systems-level change and link, where possible, to changes at the individual level.
(4) Understand that measuring successful relationship building is not about the quantity of relationships but rather about the depth of relationships and the outcomes of collaboration.
(5) Reflect on the contribution of many partners in many ways to understand the dynamics of policy change and its relationship to changes in social and cultural capital.

Does community engagement foster policy change?

Generative social capital and the resulting resilient ties that span networks create the conditions for productive discourse that develops a container for the co-construction of values, plans, and ways of working together. Respondents focused on the interactive nature of their discussions and the impact of partners seeing that their ideas and feedback were incorporated into the emerging work. This responsiveness to emerging issues and feedback is what keeps the work relevant and maintains the continuous communication loops that are necessary for success (Kania & Kramer, 2011). The process makes it possible to mobilize the "many" needed for successful policy change.

Conclusion

The Northeast Iowa FFI case offers key insights into how to manage the process of relationship building, so the relationships drive success rather than create barriers to progress. The FFI case illustrates the iterative nature of social capital development – bonding and bridging to generative – in cycles that produce new stocks of cultural capital, particularly in regard to ways of thinking and working together, and individual and collective efficacy; human capital as it relates to generating new knowledge created from place-based tacit knowing and expert knowledge; and political capital in creating understanding of how to leverage change within existing systems. The information shared by FFI members allows us to unpack the spiraling-up process and focus in on the role social capital, particularly generative social capital, plays in creating new assets that assist in changing mental models and patterns of behavior critical to effective system change and policy work.

The process of building relationships is critical to successful community and policy change work that also adheres to social justice goals. In analyzing how relationships are built in successful policy change work, the iterative and generative nature of social capital emerges as a key component in creating the momentum necessary for change efforts to persist and grow over time.

Finally, the FFI example, in keeping with work on other community change efforts, demonstrates the importance of willing investors who understand the importance of building relationships to successful community and policy change work. Investing in the groundwork that leads to strong collaborations is a long-term investment. The partners who take on this work often devote both time and energy beyond their initial commitment. Addressing the time commitment needed for relationship building remains a consistent part of the work around capacity, corroborating Kania and Kramer's thesis that it is an essential resource-intensive part of collective impact work.

Acknowledgments

The authors are indebted to the FFI leadership team for sharing their knowledge and expertise and directing us to this topic, to Amanda Malcolm for assisting with the interviews, and to the WKKF for consistent, long-term financial support of the FFI work.

References

Beck, D., & Purcell, R. (2013). *International community organising*. Bristol: Policy Press.

Bourdieu, P. (1986). The forms of capital. In J. Richardson (Ed.), *Handbook of theory for the sociology of education* (pp. 241–258). New York, NY: Greenwood.

Chazdon, S. A., & Lott, S. (2010). Ready for engagement: Using key informant interviews to measure community social capacity. *Community Development, 41*, 156–175.

Coke, T., Nielsen, S., Henry, A., Ramos, J., Seward, S., & Smith, B. (2009). Social justice. In S. Lawerence (Ed.), *Grantmaking II: An update on U.S. foundation trends* (pp.1–2). New York, NY: Foundation Center.

Coleman, J. S. (1988). Social capital in the creation of human capital. *American Journal of Sociology, 94*, S95–S120.

Cooperrider, D., Sorensen, P. Jr., Yaeger, T., & Whitney, D. (Eds.). (2001). *Appreciative inquiry: An emerging direction for organization development*. Champaign, IL: Stipes Publishing L.L.C.

Coradini, O. L. (2010). The divergences between Bourdieu's and Coleman's notions of social capital and their epistemological limits. *Social Science Information, 49*, 563–583.

des Villes-Sante, R., & Dooris, M. (2009). Community participation and empowerment in healthy cities. *Health Promotion International, 24*, 51. Retrieved from: www.heapro.oxfordjournals.org/content/24/suppl_1/i45.full

Earl, S., Carden, F., & Smutylo, T. (2001). *Outcome mapping: Building learning and reflection into development programs*. Ottowa, CA: International Development Research Centre.

Emery, M., Flora, C., Gutierrez, I., & Fernandez-Baca, E. (2006). Spiraling-up: Mapping community transformation with community capitals framework. *Community Development, 37*, 19–35.

Flora, C. B., & Flora, J. (2012). *Rural communities: Legacy & change*. Boulder, CO: Westview Press.

Fukuyama, F. (1995). Social capital and the global economy. *Foreign Affairs, 74*, 89–103.

Fulbright-Anderson, K., & Aupos, P. (2006). *Community change: Theories, practice, and evidence*. Washington, DC: The Aspen Institute.

Gittell, M., Newman, K., Bockmeyer, J., & Lindsay, R. (1998). Expanding civic opportunity: Urban empowerment zones. *Urban Affairs Review, 33*, 530–558.

Glickman, N. J., & Servon, L. J. (1998). More than bricks and sticks: Five components of community development corporation capacity. *Housing Policy Debate, 9*, 497–539.
Granovetter, M. S. (1973). The strength of weak ties. *American Journal of Sociology, 78*, 1360–1380.
Jagpal, N., & Laskowski, K. (2013). *The state of giving to underserved communities 2011*. Washington, DC: The National Committee for Responsive Philanthropy.
Kania, J., & Kramer, M. (2011). Collective impact. *Stanford Social Innovation Review, Winter*, 36–41. Retrieved from http://www.ssireview.org/pdf/2011_WI_Feature_Kania.pdf
Keating, K., & Gasteyer, S. P. (2012). The role of cultural capital in the development of community leadership: Toward an integrated program model. *Community Development, 43*, 147–168.
Kellogg Foundation. (n.d.). *W. K. Kellogg Foundation: Food and fitness*. Retrieved from http://www.activelivingbydesign.org/what-we-do/funders-initiatives/kellogg-food-fitness
Kubisch, A., Auspos, P., Brown, P., & Dewar, T. (2010). *Voices from the field III: Lessons and challenges from two decades of community change efforts*. Washington, DC: The Aspen Institute.
Lachance, L., Carpenter, L., Emery, M., & Luluquisen, M. (2014). An introduction to the Food & Fitness community partnerships and this special issue. *Community Development, 45*, 215–219.
Perkins, D., Hughey, J., & Speer, P. W. (2002). Community psychology perspectives on social capital theory and community development practice. *Community Development Society Journal, 33*, 33–52.
Popp, J., MacKean, G., Casebeer, A., Milward, H., & Lindstrom, R. (2013, July 29). *Inter-organizational networks: A critical review of the literature to inform practice*. Retrieved from http://health-leadership-research.royalroads.ca/
Portes, A. (2000). Social capital: Its origins and applications in modern sociology. In E. Lesser (Ed.), *Knowledge and social capital* (pp. 43–67). Boston, MA: Butterworth-Heinemann.
Putnam, R. D. (1995). Bowling alone: America's declining social capital. *Journal of Democracy, 6*, 65–78.
Salvador, R. (2014). True wealth. In *Keynote follow up presented at Practical Farmers of Iowa Annual Conference*, Ames, IA.
Stoecker, R. (1999). Are academics irrelevant? Roles for scholars in participatory research. *American Behavioral Scientist, 42*, 840–854.
Turner, R. S. (1999). Entrepreneurial neighborhood initiatives: Political capital in community development. *Economic Development Quarterly, 13*, 15–22.
Walzer, N. (2012). *Common elements in creative strategies for community change*. St Paul, MN: Presented to the Bush Foundation.

Moving toward and beyond equity: the Food & Fitness approach to increasing opportunities for health in communities

Laurie Lachance, Laurie Carpenter, Martha Quinn, Margaret K. Wilkin and Noreen M. Clark

Center for Managing Chronic Disease, University of Michigan, Ann Arbor, USA

Through creating avenues for authentic civic engagement of individuals living in vulnerable communities, the Food & Fitness community partnerships have actualized innovative ways to change the trajectory of health outcomes in neighborhoods across the United States. Working to increase the availability of healthy, locally grown food and opportunities for physical activity in communities that have suffered from years of disinvestment, the partnerships have moved toward and beyond merely bridging the equity gap.

Over the last few decades, the understanding of inequities related to health in populations has shifted from a focus on individuals and individual-level risk factors (Keys, 1980; Nieto, 1999) to the realization that risk is generated by conditions that influence opportunity for health (House, Schoeni, Kaplan, & Pollack, 2008; Lantz et al., 1998; Williams & Collins, 2001), and that these conditions operate at the level of neighborhoods and communities (Diez Roux, 2007; Morenoff & Lynch, 2004; Schulz et al., 2012).

Efforts to change conditions at the population level that focus only on the population as a whole can result in shifting health-related risk, but the gap, which relates to levels of individual baseline risk, and resources, does not change, and has in some instances been shown to increase due to variability in baseline risk and resources (Frohlich & Potvin, 2008; Victora, Barros, & Vaughan, 2001). However, directing efforts only toward vulnerable populations can reinforce negative stereotypes (Powell, 1999; Williams & Collins, 1995). Powell cautions that disparities in health cannot be our sole focus. Rather, the goal is to foster structures that support positive life outcomes with the ideal being universal access (Powell, 1999).

Strategies that address this equity gap, while at the same time increasing opportunities for health in the overall population, move the work beyond merely a focus on access, which is only one of many factors that constrain healthy outcomes (Frohlich & Potvin, 2008; Powell, 1999).

In order to focus efforts fostering supportive structures for positive health outcomes on both the population as a whole and on vulnerable populations, critical nuances related to health risk and efforts to create changes in opportunities for health must be considered (Frohlich & Potvin, 2008; Kuh & Ben-Shlomo, 2004; Link & Phelan, 1995; Phelan, Link, Diez-Roux, Kawachi, & Levin, 2004; Powell, 1999).

These nuances relate to underlying causes that increase an individual's vulnerability to risk, such as limited access to resources, knowledge, power, money, and beneficial social connections (Link & Phelan, 1995; Phelan et al., 2004). Attending to these nuances in an effort to reduce health risks in populations requires a consideration of two pathways: life trajectory and concentration of risk (Frohlich & Potvin, 2008; Morenoff & Lynch, 2004).

Life trajectory and the whole of life experiences determine one's position in a distribution of risk, and shifting this risk distribution requires attention to the history of life experiences (Kuh & Ben-Shlomo, 2004; Phelan et al., 2004). Efforts that do not consider life history can mask important considerations for addressing health, such as the cumulative effects of limited resources on the management of health conditions, including lack of medical care coverage and other life problems.

Consideration of concentration of risk is critical to efforts aimed at reducing health risk in populations. Those who start with lower exposures to risk at the beginning of a health-related intervention will appear to derive more benefit from the intervention than those who start with greater exposures to risk. Those who are exposed to contextual conditions that reduce opportunity for health are, for example, more likely to experience multiple morbidities, which can modify the effect of any one condition (Diez Roux, 2007; Frohlich & Potvin, 2008; Morenoff & Lynch, 2004). Thus, a one-size-fits-all approach to reducing health risk will not have the needed impact on those who are at most risk for negative health outcomes.

Life trajectory and concentration of risk are often due to a history of structural racism and community disinvestment, which must be addressed explicitly in order to shift the understanding of the process for addressing health and health-related outcomes (Kuh & Ben-Shlomo, 2004; Morenoff & Lynch, 2004). Individuals and communities suffering under structural racism often encounter multiple mechanisms and processes which interface to affect life trajectory and chances (Powell, 1999; Williams & Collins, 1995). Thinking in terms of people's life chances brings the lens closer to focusing on elements such as quality of schools and housing, neighborhood safety related to crime and drugs, and lack of infrastructure such as lighting and sidewalks. These elements are critical to include in structural change efforts aimed at improving health.

Strategies that focus on neighborhood context and create opportunities for communities to inform decision-making with respect to changes affecting health are needed. The Food & Fitness community partnerships have created a process for enlisting these strategies. Food & Fitness was conceived by the W. K. Kellogg Foundation (WKKF) as work that would focus on changing systems and infrastructures in vulnerable communities. The vision was for these changes to evolve from true civic engagement in communities that would build capacity to create change with the potential to be sustainable over time (Lachance, Carpenter, Emery, & Luluquisen, 2014). The Food & Fitness partnerships are creating change in these ways in schools and in the community related to food infrastructure and the built environment, in neighborhoods with histories of disinvestment, structural racism, and greater exposure to risk. In order to accomplish these changes, they have focused on first creating frameworks that allow for collaborative efforts that deliberately create a shared vision, assess community strengths, prioritize efforts, recruit and support youth as leaders, equip partnership members with advocacy and policy change skills, ensure that those who are in leadership positions reflect the community, monitor resources, and recruit strategic partners who can further influence the decision-making to create the needed changes.

From the start of the Food & Fitness community work, the WKKF has served as a leader and partner, shaping the overall vision and providing key technical assistance concerning the processes of creating and maintaining a shared vision within each of the sites and relationship building – key avenues for moving individuals and organizations from a focus on self-interest to common goals that serve the community in a collective way. A strong aspect of the technical assistance has been a focus on racial healing and understanding the effects of structural racism on the health of children, families, and communities. Grantees and partners have been invited to participate in deep personal work and reflection related to our country's history of racism and the influence of racism on our structures and practices that directly impact health and opportunities.

Current practices are in place in many communities – based on a history of structural racism, power dynamics based on privilege and education, and exclusionary practices – that make it difficult for the voices of those who most represent the community to be involved in the discourse about decisions being made. To shift from current practices that are based on overall population (non-individualized) approaches and service delivery to models based on ownership, recognition of the history of injustice, attention to who is engaged, and acknowledgment of power dynamics requires a systems interrupter. Systems interrupters are able to divert trajectories that have long been in place in communities, which is critical in creating the dynamic systems changes necessary for authentic transformation (Figure 1).

Examples of systems interrupters that have increased opportunities for community engagement in decision-making regarding health in the neighborhoods of the Food & Fitness community partnerships include shifting of resources to organizations and efforts that support the shared vision of the work and create economic growth at the local level. Additional examples involve strategic recruitment of individuals and organizations into

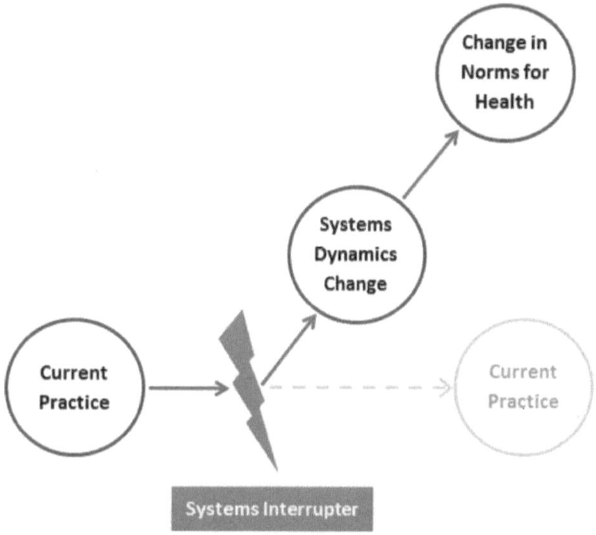

Figure 1. The Food & Fitness systems change process to increase opportunities for health in communities.

the collaborative who reflect the voices of the community and create opportunities for true discourse in the process of change.

The approach to this work was first shaped by the role of philanthropy as a partner, working with community, stepping back and listening to community voices, and facilitating capacity for community change (Doctor, 2014). With the ongoing support provided by WKKF, as well as an evaluation that has resulted in a participatory design for capturing outcomes, processes, and overall impact for the Food & Fitness community partnership work (Lachance, Carpenter, Quinn, et al., 2014), the partnerships have realized and tracked many outcomes that have empowered community members to be engaged in creating more opportunities for health: the empowerment of youth to effect change through the Food Empowerment Education and Sustainability Team (FEEST) work that has created a platform for youth-driven change related to food justice and food systems change (Charbonneau, Cheadle, Orbé, Frey, & Gaoloch, 2014); innovative methods for engagement and distribution of resources that are in line with shared community vision (Sands, Bankert, Rataj, Maitin, & Sostre, 2014); community-based participatory approaches that create collaborative structures and processes such as shared power and decision-making, which are critical to successful partnerships among diverse individuals and groups in communities (Luluquisen & Pettis, 2014); a focus on relationship building that allows for mobilizing the social capital needed to create systems change (Emery & Bregendahl, 2014); and overall attention to moving toward and beyond equity of access to the resources needed for health in communities.

Efforts to change the trajectory of health outcomes in vulnerable populations must go beyond merely bridging the gap between access of resources in the dominant culture and those most at risk, and focus on universal access to opportunities for health, while at the same time creating avenues for authentic civic engagement in subpopulations that experience higher levels of risk and lower levels of resources for health. From the beginning of the Food & Fitness work, engagement has been the driver toward change. Without the creation of authentic avenues for including voices that reflect the communities and strategic engagement across multiple sectors, sustainable changes in food systems and the built environment that positively change the trajectory of health outcomes in vulnerable communities could not occur.

The Food & Fitness partnerships are continuing to make changes in systems and infrastructures in their communities, and these changes are showing positive impacts in the lives of children and families in these communities.

Acknowledgement

We acknowledge Linda Jo Doctor for her inspiration and dedication to this work.

References

Charbonneau, D., Cheadle, A., Orbé, C., Frey, M., & Gaoloch, B. (2014). FEEST on this: Youth engagement for community change in the King County Food and Fitness Initiative. *Community Development, 45*: 3, 240–251.

Diez Roux, A. V. (2007). Neighborhoods and health: Where are we and were do we go from here? *Revue d'Épidémiologie et de Santé Publique, 55*, 13–21.

Doctor, L. J. (2014). Philanthropy's role: Working alongside communities to support social change. *Community Development, 45*: 3, 220–226.

Emery, M., & Bregendahl, C. (2014). Speaking truth: The art, craft, and context for building the trust and relationships necessary to undertake system change. *Community Development, 45*, 277–290.

Frohlich, K. L., & Potvin, L. (2008). Transcending the known in public health practice. *American Journal of Public Health, 98*, 216–221.
House, J. S., Schoeni, R. F., Kaplan, G. A., & Pollack, H. (2008). The health effects of social and economic policy: The promise and challenge for research and policy. In R. Schoeni, J. S. House, G. A. Kaplan, & H. Pollack (Eds.), *Making Americans healthier: Social and economic policy as health policy* (pp. 3–26). New York, NY: Russell Sage Foundation.
Keys, A. B. (1980). *Seven countries: A multivariate analysis of death and coronary heart disease.* Cambridge, MA: Harvard University Press.
Kuh, D., & Ben-Shlomo, Y. (2004). *A life course approach to chronic diseases epidemiology.* New York, NY: Oxford University Press.
Lachance, L., Carpenter, L., Emery, M., & Luluquisen, M. (2014). An introduction to the Food & Fitness community partnerships and this special issue. *Community Development, 45*, 215–219.
Lachance, L., Carpenter, L., Quinn, M., Wilkin, M. K., Green, E., Tsuchiya, K. … Clark, N. M. (2014). Food & Community: The cross-site evaluation of the W. K. Kellogg Foundation Food & Fitness community partnerships. *Community Development, 45*, 227–239.
Lantz, P. M., House, J. S., Lepkowski, J. M., Williams, D. R., Mero, R. P., & Chen, J. (1998). Socioeconomic factors, health behaviors, and mortality. *JAMA, 279*, 1703–1708.
Link, B. G., & Phelan, J. C. (1995). Social conditions as fundamental causes of disease. *Journal of Health and Social Behavior, 35*, 80–94.
Luluquisen, M., & Pettis, L. (2014). Community engagement for policy and systems change. *Community Development, 45*, 252–262.
Morenoff, J. D., & Lynch, J. W. (2004). What makes a place healthy? Neighborhood influence on racial/ethnic disparities in health over the life course. In N. B. Anderson, R. A. Bulatao, & B. Cohen (Eds.), *Critical perspectives on racial and ethnic differences in health in late life* (pp. 406–449). Washington, DC: The National Academies Press.
Nieto, F. J. (1999). Cardiovascular disease and risk factor epidemiology: A look back at the epidemic of the 20th century. *American Journal of Public Health, 89*, 292–294.
Phelan, J. C., Link, B. G., Diez-Roux, A., Kawachi, I., & Levin, B. (2004). "Fundamental causes" of social inequalities in mortality: A test of the theory. *Journal of Health and Social Behavior, 45*, 265–285.
Powell, J. A. (1999). Race, poverty, and urban sprawl: Access to opportunities through regional strategies. *Forum for Social Economics, 28*, 1–20.
Sands, C. H., Bankert, S. C., Rataj, S., Maitin, M., & Sostre, J. (2014). "Call for Partnerships": An innovative strategy to establish grassroots partnerships to transform the food and fitness environments. *Community Development, 45*, 263–278.
Schulz, A. J., Mentz, G., Lachance, L., Johnson, J., Gaines, C., & Israel, B. A. (2012). Associations between socioeconomic status and allostatic load: Effects of neighborhood poverty. *American Journal of Public Health, 102*, 1706–1714.
Victora, C. G., Barros, F. C., & Vaughan, J. P. (2001). The impact of health interventions on inequalities: Infant and child health in Brazil. In D. Leon, & G. Walt (Eds.), *Poverty, inequality, and health* (pp. 125–136). Oxford: Oxford University Press.
Williams, D. R., & Collins, C. (1995). US socioeconomic and racial differences in health: Patterns and explanations. *Annual Review of Sociology, 21*, 349–386.
Williams, D. R., & Collins, C. (2001). Racial residential segregation: A fundamental cause of racial disparities in health. *Public Health Reports, 116*, 404–416.

Index

Note: Page numbers followed by 'f' refer to figures and followed by 't' refer to tables.